MODERN GERIATRICS SERIES

Series Editor: J. Wedgwood

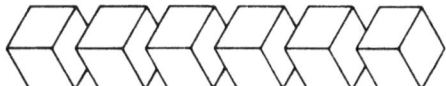

INFECTIONS IN THE ELDERLY

MODERN GERIATRICS SERIES

Series Editor: J. Wedgwood

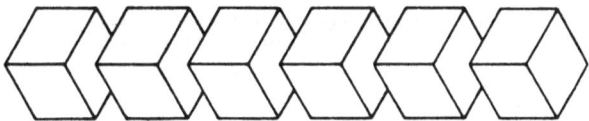

INFECTIONS IN THE ELDERLY

Edited by Michael J. Denham

Department of Geriatric Medicine
Northwick Park Hospital and Clinical Research Centre, Harrow

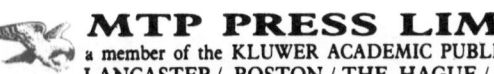 **MTP PRESS LIMITED**
a member of the KLUWER ACADEMIC PUBLISHERS GROUP
LANCASTER / BOSTON / THE HAGUE / DORDRECHT

Published in the UK and Europe by
MTP Press Limited
Falcon House
Lancaster, England

British Library Cataloguing in Publication Data

Infections in the elderly. – (Modern geriatrics series)
1. Aged – Diseases   2. Communicable diseases
I. Denham, Michael J.   II. Series
618.97'69   RC112

Published in the USA by
MTP Press
A division of Kluwer Boston Inc
190 Old Derby Street
Hingham, MA 02043, USA

Library of Congress Cataloging-in-Publication Data

Main entry under title:

Infections in the elderly.

(Modern geriatrics series)
Includes bibliographies and index.
1. Bacterial diseases.   2. Aged – Diseases.
3. Virus diseases.   4 Infection – Age factors.
I. Denham, Michael J. (Michael John)   II. Series.
[DNLM: 1. Communicable Diseases – in old age.
WC 100 I40242]
RC115.I526   1985   618.97'69   85-24111
ISBN-13: 978-94-010-8334-8   e-ISBN-13: 978-94-009-4135-9
DOI: 10.1007/978-94-009-4135-9

Typesetting by:
BPCC Northern Printers Ltd.
Northgate, Blackburn

Contents

List of Contributors

R. J. ANGUS
Department of Geriatric Medicine
Northwick Park Hospital and
 Clinical Research Centre
Watford Road
Harrow
Middlesex HA1 3UJ
ENGLAND

F. D. BEGGS
Department of General Surgery
Northwick Park Hospital and
 Clinical Research Centre
Watford Road
Harrow
Middlesex HA1 3UJ
ENGLAND

M. J. CLARKE-WILLIAMS
Consultant Physician in Geriatric
 Medicine
Portsmouth and South East
 Hampshire Health District
Queen Alexandra Hospital
Cosham
Portsmouth PO6 3LY
ENGLAND

M. J. DENHAM
Department of Geriatric Medicine
Northwick Park Hospital and
 Clinical Research Centre
Watford Road
Harrow
Middlesex HA1 3UJ
ENGLAND

R. A. FOX
Department of Medicine
 (Geriatrics)
Dalhousie University
Camp Hill Hospital
Robie Street
Halifax, Nova Scotia
CANADA B3H 3G2

S. K. GOOLAMALI
Department of Dermatology
Northwick Park Hospital and
 Clinical Research Centre
Watford Road
Harrow
Middlesex HA1 3UJ
ENGLAND

B. E. JUEL-JENSEN
Nuffield Department of Medicine
University of Oxford
John Radcliffe Hospital
Headington
Oxford OX3 9DU
ENGLAND

A. E. KARK
Department of Surgery
Northwick Park Hospital and
 Clinical Research Centre
Watford Road
Harrow
Middlesex HA1 3UJ
ENGLAND

J. E. KASIK
Department of Internal Medicine
College of Medicine, University of
  Iowa VAMC Iowa City
IA 52242
USA

B. MOORE-SMITH
Department of Geriatric Medicine
Ipswich Hospital
Heath Road
Ipswich
Suffolk IP4 5PD
ENGLAND

M. F. MUHLEMANN
Department of Dermatology
Central Middlesex Hospital
Acton Lane
London NW10 7NS
ENGLAND

T. E. A PETO
Nuffield Department of Medicine
University of Oxford
John Radcliffe Hospital
Headington
Oxford OX3 9DU
ENGLAND

P. J. SANDERSON
Department of Microbiology
Edgeware General Hospital
Edgeware
Middlesex HA8 0AD
ENGLAND

H. SMITH
Lister Unit
Northwick Park Hospital and
  Clinical Research Centre
Watford Road
Harrow
Middlesex HA1 3UJ
ENGLAND

R. K. T. WILLIAMS
Department of Geriatric Medicine
Dorset County Hospital
Dorchester
Dorset DT1 1TS
ENGLAND

Preface

Public health and antiseptic measures, vaccination and antibiotics, have all contributed to the reduction in the incidence and impact of diseases due to infections in younger age groups. Unfortunately, however, infections remain a very important cause of both morbidity and mortality in the elderly.

The reasons for the continued effect of infection on the older person are multifactorial. Firstly, the immune response alters with age and may result in opportunistic infections. Secondly, while the diagnosis and management of some infections in the elderly can present little problem, altered signs and symptoms in other older patients, especially the old elderly, can cause considerable diagnostic difficulties with resulting delays in definitive treatment. Thirdly, a degree of complacency can develop because some infections are seldom seen and, consequently, may not be considered in the differential diagnosis. The presence of other, more common, diseases serve only to distract attention and confuse the diagnosis. Since the number of elderly people is increasing, the need for continued high standard of skill in diagnosis and management is emphasized.

These factors are considered in this book by contributors who are experienced in their fields. The altered immune response with age, the appropriate use of antibiotics in older people and the latest developments of therapy are reviewed. Infections in various body systems are considered, with emphasis on differing presentations and diagnostic difficulties, ways of improving diagnostic skills as well as management and treatment. The subject material should therefore be of value to all those who treat elderly people, both in the community and in hospital.

Michael J. Denham

Series Editor's Note

This series attempts to keep abreast of developments in Geriatric Medicine. This is no easy task in such a rapidly expanding subject.

The editors of each volume and their authors have approached the subject from the point of view of practising clinicians, experienced in what can now be called the British tradition of Geriatric Medicine. The text is aimed at those wishing to acquire a more specialized knowledge of Geriatric Medicine either in hospital or in general practice. At the same time it is hoped that it will be of value to both undergraduate and postgraduate students.

Nevertheless, it has been said that we 'all practise geriatrics now', and, bearing in mind the kernel of truth in this observation, it is hoped that this series will be of interest to an even wider medical readership.

The Series Editor has always favoured a multi-disciplinary approach to training in Geriatric Medicine, and hopes that this slant will also allow the Series to be of value to our colleagues in the para-medical and nursing professions.

The first volume deals with acute geriatric medicine, a subject which has become of particular importance with the emergency admission policies of a number of geriatric units today, and the combination of general and general medical 'firms'.

The second volume deals with the difficult problem of fits, faints and falls in the old.

The third volume is about infections in the elderly.

John Wedgwood, MA, MD, FRCP

1

The Principles of Antibiotic Practice in the Elderly

P. J. SANDERSON

INTRODUCTION

Antibiotic practice is a changing scene. Many different drugs have become available since penicillin and the sulphonamides were discovered and new agents continue to appear. Indeed, antibacterials with novel molecules and properties are still in the developmental stage and it will be of great interest to see whether or not they establish a clinical role. Equally, bacteria have successfully survived the antibiotic era and changing patterns of antibiotic resistance demand greater accuracy in antibiotic prescribing. In some infections established antibiotics continue to be drugs of choice, but new drug regimens and new antibiotic combinations for seriously ill patients are being investigated.

This chapter discusses the principles of antibiotic use and comments on methods of bacterial diagnosis. The main groups of antibacterials are described, together with their interaction with other drugs, use in impaired renal function, and future developments.

USE OF ANTIBIOTICS

Appropriate Prescriptions

Surveys in hospitals have demonstrated that doctors frequently prescribe antibiotics without being aware of the type of bacteria they are treating [1], and sometimes little effort has been made to determine the site of infection.

1

A careful history and usually an examination of the patient, as well as the careful collection of specimens, are prerequisites for any antibiotic prescription. If the presence of infection seems uncertain, as may be the case more often in elderly patients than in the younger patients, it may be appropriate to obtain bacteriological samples and re-examine the patient with the available results the next day. If an antibiotic prescription is justified treatment should begin without delay, but not before specimens have been taken. The overriding determinant of the 'best guess' choice of antibiotic will be the site of infection and the type of bacteria associated with it, taking into account previous infections and antibiotic therapy, renal function and concurrent antibiotics. It is useful to recall the type of bacteria associated with different sites of infection (Table 1.1).

Table 1.1   Bacteria associated with different sites of infection

Site of infection	Common bacterial pathogens
Blood	*Escherichia coli* other coliforms *Staphylococcus aureus* streptococci – *Strep. pneumoniae* β-haemolytic streptococci
Urinary tract	*Escherichia coli* other coliforms enterococci staphylococci
Bones and joints	*Staphylococcus aureus*
Soft tissue	Streptococcus group A *Staphylococcus aureus*
Abdominal abscess	coliforms anaerobes less common: *Staph. aureus* enterococci *Strep. milleri*
Liver abscess	anaerobes *Streptococcus milleri* coliforms
Lung	*Streptococcus pneumoniae* *Haemophilus influenzae* *Mycoplasma pneumoniae* less common: *Staph. aureus* *Klebsiella* spp. *Legionella* spp.
Upper respiratory tract (sinusitis, otitis media)	*Streptococcus pneumoniae* *Haemophilus influenzae*
Throat	Streptococcus group A

Although the appropriate doses and duration of treatment in many infections are uncertain (Table 1.2), it is logical from the point of view of bacterial resistance to expose the patient, the pathogen and normal bacterial flora of the patient to the least total amount of antibiotic commensurate with efficacy. This means that adequate doses must be given so that therapeutic concentrations are reached at the site of infection. Prescriptions should, in general, give high doses for short periods of time since this will reverse the infectious processes quickly and expose the bacterial flora to less antibiotic.

Table 1.2 Appropriate antibiotics for initial treatment of different infections (that is, specimens for microbiology already taken but results awaited) (To correlate with Table 1.1)

Infection	Antibiotics
Septicaemia	gentamicin (i.v.) plus piperacillin (i.v.) (or azlocillin or ticarcillin or cefuroxime) plus metronidazole (i.v. or oral or rectal) or cefuroxime (i.v.) or ceftazidime (i.v.) alone or with metronidazole
Urinary infection	co-trimoxazole nitrofurantoin nalidixic acid ampicillin/amoxycillin
Osteomyelitis, septic arthritis	flucloxacillin (i.v.) plus fucidin (i.v. or oral)
Soft tissue infection, including cellulitis	benzyl penicillin (i.v.) plus flucloxacillin (i.v.) (erythromycin, cefuroxime or clindamycin in penicillin-sensitive patients)
Abdominal sepsis (peritonitis and abscess)	as for septicaemia
Cholangitis	cefuroxime (i.v. or i.m.) or ampicillin/amoxycillin (i.v. or i.m.) plus gentamicin (i.v. or i.m.) plus metronidazole (oral or rectal)
Liver abscess	benzyl penicillin (i.v.) plus gentamicin or cefuroxime (i.v.) plus metronidazole (i.v.)
Bronchitis, acute exacerbation of chronic obstructive airways disease	first choice: ampicillin/amoxycillin (confirm sensitivities of organisms) second choice: co-trimoxazole or erythromycin or augmentin
Pneumonia	
community-acquired	as for bronchitis
hospital-acquired	cefuroxime
atypical	erythromycin
Upper respiratory tract infection	amoxycillin or co-trimoxazole
Sore throat	penicillin or amoxycillin (for 10–14 days)
Meningitis	chloramphenicol (i.v.)

Routes of Administration

It is more comfortable for a patient to receive drugs by mouth rather than by injection. Nevertheless, absorption of many antibiotics from the intestinal tract is poor and even that of agents specially formulated for this route, such as flucloxacillin, amoxycillin and erythromycin stearate, is incomplete. In many cases it will be beneficial to institute therapy by intramuscular or intravenous routes for the first 48 hours or several days and then to continue therapy orally. The advent of peripheral intravenous catheters has made the intravenous administration of antibiotics much easier, and slow bolus injection is safe with penicillins, cephalosporins and aminoglycosides. Bolus injections will give immediate high blood levels which rapidly decline during the first half hour in the 'phase of distribution'; subsequently, serum levels decline less rapidly during the 'phase of equilibriation'. The penicillins and cephalosporins are excreted rapidly through the kidney and high peak concentrations of these drugs will be safe; for aminoglycosides the therapeutic range is narrow and blood levels need to be monitored. Antibiotics should be given singly, without being mixed with other antibiotics or other drugs for the intravenous or intramuscular routes. Appropriate carrier fluids can be determined from the 'insert' literature. Most antibiotics should be used immediately after their solution, but some may be retained at +4 °C for a day and, in the case of oral vancomycin, for longer.

Frequency of Dosage

Antibacterial agents are almost all excreted fairly rapidly, so that in the interval between doses most of the drug will have been excreted via the kidney or metabolized in the liver. Consequently, the concentrations of drug available at the site of infection towards the end of the interval between doses will be low, usually below the concentration required to inhibit or kill the infecting organism. In the case of penicillins and cephalosporins this could be an advantage, for surviving bacteria may regrow and again become susceptible to these antibiotics before the next dose is due. However, in the case of antibiotics that do not act on the cell wall this argument would not hold, and no scientific evidence has been adduced for this theory in penicillin therapy. It remains undecided whether a continuous concentration of antibiotic in the tissues is a more effective mode of therapy than the rising and falling levels of intermittent therapy. It is known that tissue levels in organs well supplied by blood closely follow serum levels with only slightly delayed lag times. On the other hand, antibiotic levels in body secretions, endolymph and the fluids of the eye are lower and delayed. It is uncertain, also, by how much the antibiotic level achieved at the site of infection should be higher than the concentration required to kill the organism. It is recommended in treating endocarditis, for example, that the trough level of antibiotic should be four times higher than the minimal bactericidal level. This may not always be achievable but it is known that subinhibitory concentrations of antibiotic do damage bacteria and may reduce their pathogenicity by also damaging physiological processes such as bacterial adhesion to surfaces. In summary, it would seem wise not to prolong unduly the intervals between antibiotic doses, and to achieve high peak levels.

Dosage of Antibiotics

There are three characteristics of elderly patients that may affect the amount of antibiotic they should receive: (1) they tend to have a lower body weight and reduced muscle mass in comparison with younger patients, upon whom the normal dosage range is based; (2) there may be reduced renal and liver function; (3) elderly patients are frequently prescribed more than one drug.

The serum urea or creatinine concentration may not reflect the degree of renal dysfunction that is often present in very elderly patients. The reduced muscle mass yields smaller amounts of creatinine than in younger patients and, together with a degree of defective renal tubular exchange, elderly patients may maintain an apparently normal excretion rate of serum urea and creatinine in the presence of a glomerular filtration rate of 50 ml/min. In practice the assay of serum gentamicin levels may indicate reduced renal function with more sensitivity than serum urea or creatinine, and dosage adjustment of aminoglycosides will be required more frequently in elderly patients. As an example of reduced excretion of an antibiotic in the presence of normal urea and creatinine values, it was found [2] that the serum half-life of amoxycillin in four elderly female patients was 2.7 hours, compared to 1.05 hours in younger volunteers.

Other antibiotics, for example, erythromycin, co-trimoxazole, tetracyclines and chloramphenicol, are metabolized partially or wholly in the liver, but some of the unaltered drug, together with some of the breakdown products, may be excreted by the kidney. Liver function in the elderly may also be reduced – for example, the half-life of phenylbutazone and antipyrine is lengthened in older patients. The intravenous administration of sodium fusidate (fucidin) in patients over 60 years may result in altered liver function [3], but this is probably not of clinical significance.

In infections of the kidney slow excretion may justify larger doses in order to obtain appropriate urine concentrations. In severe infections an initial loading dose of antibiotics, including aminoglycosides, will be widely distributed in the body and will not by itself lead to drug toxicity, even in the presence of renal failure.

INTERACTION OF ANTIBIOTICS WITH OTHER DRUGS

The possibility of drug interactions is increased in elderly patients, who may be receiving more than one treatment. Antibiotics affect the activity of other drugs by (1) alterations of the intestinal bacterial flora, (2) competition for serum protein carrier sites, (3) interaction with liver enzymes, and (4) competition for tubular secretion in the kidney.

Antibiotics and Blood Coagulation

Many antibiotics exert profound changes on the bacteria of the bowel leading to reduced manufacture of vitamin K and incidentally, when diarrhoea occurs, to loss of absorption of drugs given orally. The administration of vitamin K returns prothrombin times to normal, but this problem is accentuated if the patient is already on warfarin or related anticoagulants where the prothrombin time may be further lengthened.

Anticoagulation may also be affected by antibiotic competition with warfarin for serum protein carrier sites. Warfarin is 97% bound to plasma albumin and the anticoagulant effect of the remaining 3% can be increased by the release of only a small amount of the bound drug, for example when sulphonamides and nalidixic acid compete for protein carrier sites[4]. Although penicillins, and particularly flucloxacillin, are highly bound to serum proteins, they do not seem to have been associated with this effect.

Some cephalosporins have been associated recently with a disorder of coagulation. This has been attributed to the tetrathiozole ring on the side chains of latamoxef (Moxalactam), cephamandole and cefoperazone. This substance may interfere with the synthesis of prothrombin [5], and in the case of latamoxef there have been reports of significant bleeding after operations where this cephalosporin was used for prophylaxis.

Inhibition of the hepatic metabolism of warfarin has been associated with metronidazole, co-trimoxazole and chloramphenicol, increasing the patient's response to anticoagulation. On the other hand, rifampicin induces hepatic microsomal enzymes involved in the breakdown of anticoagulant; as a result stopping rifampicin may increase the patient's response to warfarin.

There may also be a direct effect by some antibacterials on platelets, and bleeding times may be prolonged in this way by chloramphenicol and co-trimoxazole. Very high doses of penicillins have been associated with a disturbance of platelet function, and for some ureidopenicillins this may persist after drug withdrawal perhaps by an effect on megakaryocytes. In summary, it is wise to monitor the prothrombin ratios of patients receiving warfarin and antibacterials at the same time.

Interaction with Diuretics

Interactions between antibiotics and diuretics are also relevant in elderly patients who are more likely to be given both agents and who have a raised incidence of renal dysfunction. Although cephalosporins are not nephrotoxic when used alone, except cephaloridine which should not now be used, in combination with diuretics they may be so. This is probably not a marked effect, but it is worth monitoring the serum creatinine in these circumstances. Similarly, ethacrynic acid and frusemide should be avoided when aminoglycosides are prescribed as they will potentiate the risk of deafness and vestibular toxicity, as they may with erythromycin. The combination of cephalosporins with aminoglycosides also carries the risk of increased nephrotoxicity, but presumably this is more likely if diuretics are also given.

Oral Hypoglycaemics

Another effect of competition for serum protein carrier sites, which is probably less clinically important but worth noting, is that some sulphonamides may increase the free, unbound sulphonylurea serum concentration by this mechanism, resulting in hypoglycaemia.

The antibacterials metabolized in the liver, mentioned above under interaction with warfarin, may also decrease the liver breakdown of tolbutamide.

Interactions during Renal Excretion

Probenecid competes with penicillins and cephalosporins for tubular excretion and enhances the serum concentrations of these drugs. Probenecid may also displace these antibiotics from serum albumin carrier sites and decrease biliary excretion. Cerebrospinal fluid concentrations are elevated because excretion through the choroid plexus is reduced.

Direct Interaction

Gentamicin may inactivate carbenicillin and ticarcillin, as well as probably other penicillins, when mixed together in a syringe or infusion. There is a possibility that this inactivation may occur in the serum, but it is unlikely to be clinically significant. Heparin may combine with aminoglycosides and inactivate them, and heparin used to maintain patency of peripheral catheters should be washed out before giving gentamicin. Blood samples for gentamicin assay should never be taken through the giving port of a peripheral needle or a cannula for this reason, and because spuriously high levels may be found from remnants of the previous injection of gentamicin.

ANTIBIOTICS AND RENAL FAILURE

Renal failure should present little difficulty to antibiotic therapy but will increase the need for monitoring serum levels. In mild forms of renal failure (creatinine clearance 50–80ml/min) only aminoglycosides, tetracyclines, vancomycin and amphotericin require changes in their dosage schedules.

Moderate creatinine clearances of 10–50ml/min require little or no adjustment of penicillins and cephalosporins, or of those drugs which are predominantly excreted via the liver, such as metronidazole, co-trimoxazole, erythromycin, chloramphenicol and fusidic acid. Gentamicin and other aminoglycosides will require close monitoring, as they should in any case in every patient over the age of 65. In this degree of renal failure tetracyclines and nitrofurantoin should be avoided or severely curtailed, only doxycycline can escape this stricture. Patients on methenamine mandelate require reduction of dosage, and chloramphenicol and colistin should be reduced or avoided. In severe renal failure, with creatinine clearances of less than 10ml/min, tetracyclines and nitrofurantoin must not be prescribed. Even at these levels of renal function, however, penicillins will continue to be excreted provided urine is produced, and as an approximate guide, doses of these drugs should be halved. Antibiotics excreted through the liver will need to be reduced also, as their breakdown products may be handled in the kidney (Table 1.3).

Table 1.3   Antibiotic dose interval in renal failure[a] (interval in hours)

| | | Creatinine clearance | | |
	Normal	50–80 ml/min	10–50 ml/min	< 10 ml/min
Penicillin-type drugs				
benzylpenicillin	4 or 6	6	6	12
cloxacillin	6	6	6	12
ampicillin	6	6	6	12
carbenicillin	6	6	6	12
Erythromycin	6	6	6	12
Sulphadimidine	6	6	12	24
Co-trimoxazole	12	12	24	48
Tetracyclines[b]	6	avoid	avoid	avoid
Doxycycline	24	24	24	48
Clindamycin	6	6	6	12
Fusidic acid	8	8	8	12
Cephaloridine	6	12	avoid	avoid
Cephazolin	6	6	12	24
Cephalexin	6	6	12	24
Chloramphenicol	6	6	12	avoid
Gentamicin[c]	6	6–12	12–24	48

[a] Partly from Bennett *et al.*[6] and Sharpstone[7]
[b] Nephrotoxic (see text)
[c] Assay serum concentrations routinely

NB: Colistin, methenamine mandelate, nitrofurantoin and vancomycin require severe reduction in dosage in the presence of any degree of renal failure (see text).

SIDE-EFFECTS OF ANTIBACTERIALS

Some side-effects will have been discussed in the previous sections on drug interactions and use in renal failure. The heavy use of antibiotics is a reflection of their safety, but side-effects occur both in the patient and in bacteria, by generating bacterial resistance.

Side-effects of Different Drug Groups

Hypersensitivity reactions to penicillins may be due to contaminants from the process of manufacture, from degradation products, particularly penicil-loyl derivatives, or from polymerization of penicillin in solution. In the latter case, the polymer may act as a haptene and combine with preformed antibody. Serum sickness reactions may also occur. Confirmation of penicillin hypersensitivity is difficult and available methods are not practicable or are unreliable. A careful history should be taken of the circumstances of the drug reaction; the patient may ascribe to penicillin a non-specific reaction, and occasionally an irrelevant symptom is attributed cautiously to penicillin by a medical adviser.

There appear to be fewer hypersensitivity reactions to the cephalosporins, and cross-sensitivity between penicillins and cephalosporins is only 8%.

The ototoxic affect of aminoglycosides is well known, but these agents are also nephrotoxic, and their combination with diuretics or cephalosporins may lead to increasing serum creatinine levels. With gentamicin the therapeutic ratio lies between a trough of 2.5mg/l and peak levels of 8–10mg/l. The ototoxic effect of gentamicin, tobramycin and netilmicin affects mainly the sense of balance while amikacin and kanamycin affect hearing particularly. These effects tend to improve on stopping the aminoglycoside, and while the vestibular damage may be compensated for to some extent, any permanent loss of hearing cannot be. It is possible that elderly patients are more sensitive to these side-effects than are younger patients.

Erythromycin may cause nausea and vomiting. The estolate is associated with liver toxicity to a greater extent than the stearate, although it is better absorbed from the gut. Rarely, erythromycin may cause deafness. Intramuscular preparations are not available, and administration via a peripheral vein very frequently causes local thrombophlebitis.

Nitrofurantoin and nalidixic acid may also cause nausea, and the former agent is associated with peripheral neuropathy following long-term administration; allergic reactions and pulmonary infiltration occur rarely. Nalidixic acid may lead to photosensitization and visual disturbances.

In co-trimoxazole most side-effects will be due to the sulphonamide component. Haemolytic anaemia may be precipitated in patients with glucose 6-phosphate dehydrogenase (G6PD) deficiency, and this may be seen also with nitrofurantoin and nalidixic acid. The Stevens–Johnson syndrome has been attributed to sulphonamides. Trimethoprim may also give rise to skin rashes but less frequently than sulphonamides. In longer-term treatment with co-trimoxazole the possibility of folate deficiency is unlikely in anyone with a normal diet, but should be considered where this is in question.

Bacterial Resistance

Antibiotics exert a selective pressure for resistance on both the pathogen and the normal flora of the human body. Resistant strains of either category will survive during antibiotic therapy and may be stimulated to transfer their antibiotic resistances by plasmids to other bacteria, including potential pathogens. *Haemophilus influenzae* now shows beta-lactamase production and consequent resistance to amoxycillin, in some 5–20% of strains. This is due to a plasmid gene possibly acquired from a resistant *Escherichia coli*. Amoxycillin will therefore be ineffective in treating pulmonary infections with these strains. There is evidence of increasing resistance to penicillin by *Streptococcus pneumoniae,* and strains resistant to high levels of penicillin and many other antibiotics have been isolated in Australia, South Africa and, on rare occasions, in North America. These strains are not yet a practical problem in Europe but all isolated strains should be tested for penicillin sensitivity in the laboratory. Meningococcal meningitis can no longer be treated initially with sulphonamides due to resistance among the different serotypes. Indeed, the sensitivity of *Neisseria meningitidis* to penicillins could be under threat, in the same way that *Neisseria gonorrhoeae* acquired penicillin resistance from a gene coding for beta-lactamase production acquired via a plasmid form *Escherichia coli*. Two approaches help to prevent antibiotic resistance: (1) careful prescribing; and (2) the early detection of resistant bacteria, followed by the isolation of patients with such organisms to prevent cross-infection. The main areas of careless use of antibiotics are: unnecessary prescriptions, unjustifiably prolonged courses of treatment and prophylaxis, topical use of antibiotics, and low doses leading to slow resolution of infection.

USES OF SPECIFIC ANTIBIOTICS

Penicillins

Penicillin and Flucloxacillin

These antibiotics are characterized by their safety, and have few side-effects apart from hypersensitivity. They are excreted rapidly through the kidney, the half-life of benzylpenicillin being 25 min. Penicillin will inhibit and kill pneumococci, streptococci, *Neisseria meningitidis* and sensitive strains of staphylococci (only some 10% of the total) at lower concentrations than any other antibiotic. Unfortunately, the absorption of oral penicillins is poor and high doses should be given.

Flucloxacillin resists beta-lactamases and is the drug of choice for most strains of *Staphylococcus aureus*. Preferably, this drug should be used for the oral route, and cloxacillin used intramuscularly or intravenously, since it is more active but absorbed from the gut more poorly.

Amoxycillin and Ampicillin

Amoxycillin and esters of ampicillin show improved intestinal absorption over ampicillin itself, and this is an advantage which may be worth their increased cost. Amoxycillin has also been shown to penetrate sputum in higher amounts than ampicillin and to kill bacteria *in vitro* more quickly than ampicillin. These antibiotics are inactivated by beta-lactamases of *Staph. aureus*, many coliforms and most *Bacteroides* spp. They remain the drugs of choice for *H. influenzae* chest infections, provided the strain is beta-lactamase-negative, and for enterococcal (*Streptococcus faecalis*) endocarditis.

Ureidopenicillins

The ureidopenicillins, namely ticarcillin, azlocillin and piperacillin, show broad-spectrum activity against Gram-negative bacilli and *Pseudomonas* spp. but remain susceptible to the beta-lactamases mentioned above. Ticarcillin is a disodium salt and the recommended dose of 20 g a day for a pseudomonas infection carries with it about 60 mEq of sodium ion; the sodium load of azlocillin and piperacillin is half of this, being monosodium salts. Hypokalaemia may also occur with these agents.

Augmentin

Two new pharmacological discoveries relate to the penicillins. Clavulanic acid is a weak antibiotic able to combine strongly with, and immobilize, beta-lactamases. Given in combination with amoxycillin, as augmentin, it exhibits similar pharmacological properties to amoxycillin and penetrates body compartments to a similar extent. At the site of infection beta-lactamases produced by an invading organism are removed by clavulanic acid, allowing amoxycillin to be active. At present, the clinical role of augmentin is still being assessed; it may be useful in *H. influenzae* chest infection and in upper respiratory tract infection. It is being advocated for soft tissue infections and in abdominal infections where it is active against beta-lactamase producing *Staph. aureus* and *Bacteroides fragilis,* respectively. However, augmentin will have to compete with other well-established and effective agents already available for these situations.

Aztreonam

The second development is the discovery of a radical variation of the basic penicillin molecule. The natural production by *Chromobacterium violacium* of the beta-lactam portion of the penicillin molecule, without the five-membered thiozolidine portion, has been exploited in the commercial production of monobactams, with side-chain substitutions at three of the four member sites. The first clinically available monobactam, aztreonam, will soon be marketed. This agent is more resistant to beta-lactamases than the broad-spectrum penicillins and has wide activity against coliforms and *Pseudomonas* spp., but is inactive against Gram-positive organisms. With this spectrum, and with the safety of the penicillins, this antibiotic may herald the successful replacement of aminoglycosides.

Cephalosporins

These drugs resemble the penicillins by possessing a four-membered beta-lactam ring joined to a six-membered thiazine ring; they act on the bacterial cell wall in a similar way but resist a wider range of beta-lactamases. Cephalosporins show good activity against coliforms, streptococci, and *Staph. aureus,* but only ceftazidime is active against pseudomonas. They are safe, and hypersensitivity reactions are possibly less frequent than for penicillins.

The broad activity and lack of side-effects of cephalosporins are particularly advantageous in elderly patients for serious, undiagnosed infection. The loss of renal function occurring with age, which may not be sufficient to alter serum creatinine and urea measurement, will not affect excretion of these drugs as it may aminoglycosides. In more severe degrees of renal failure these agents will be safer and easier to use than aminoglycosides. Close monitoring of serum concentrations is not required and high peak levels can be assured by adequate doses; nephrotoxicity is unlikely when the modern cephalosporins are used alone.

Cefuroxime, Ceftazidime and Cefotaxime

Cefuroxime is useful in hospital-acquired chest infection in elderly patients, where its activity against pneumococci, *H. influenzae* and possible but unlikely coliform chest infections is greater than that of amoxycillin. Cef-tazidime has a somewhat wider spectrum of activity than cefuroxime, extended to pseudomonas, whereas cefotaxime is less reliable against the latter organism. Oral forms of cephalosporins are less valuable and their role in general is restricted. Cephalosporins are more frequently associated with pseudomembranous colitis than are aminoglycosides. The onset of diar-rhoea in any patient while on antibiotics should be investigated with this diagnosis in mind.

Aminoglycosides

Gentamicin, Tobramycin, Netilmicin and Amikacin

Gentamicin is a well-established and efficient antibiotic when properly used. The narrow therapeutic range demands regular assay of serum levels, par-ticularly in elderly patients where renal dysfunction is more common. Tob-ramycin is more active against pseudomonas and netilmicin is possibly less toxic than gentamicin, but both are otherwise very similar to gentamicin and require monitoring of serum levels. Many hospitals hold amikacin in reserve for gentamicin-resistant organisms.

Aminoglycosides, it should be remembered, are not broad-spectrum agents, being active against coliforms and pseudomonas and inactive against Gram-positive cocci (except *Staph. aureus)* and anaerobic bacteria.

Erythromycin and Clindamycin

Erythromycin has two main uses; first, as an agent of choice for *Staph. aureus* and streptococci in patients who are hypersensitive to penicillins. Erythromycin is also a useful first-line agent in chest infections since it is active against *H. influenzae* (both beta-lactamase producers and non-producers), as well as pneumococci, *Mycoplasma pneumoniae* and *Chlamydia psittaci,* and it is the antibiotic choice for Legionnaire's disease. If the history of the patient reveals a possible exposure to these agents, or the patient is non-responsive to appropriate doses of ampicillin or amoxycillin, erythromycin would be an appropriate choice. Gastrointestinal absorption of erythromycin stearate is poor, and doses of 2 or 3 g daily should be given.

Clindamycin has high activity against *Staph. aureus* and other Gram-positive organisms, and it remains a useful agent for these organisms when penicillins, erythromycin or co-trimoxazole cannot be used. The association of clindamycin with pseudomembranous colitis has led to restricted use, but when the drug is indicated this should not be a deterrent. Apart from this complication, clindamycin appears to be a safe antibacterial which pene-trates deep infections well.

Co-trimoxazole

This combination of sulphamethoxazole and trimethoprim has been a successful one for treating urinary tract and respiratory infections. It is now thought, however, that the marked *in vitro* synergistic effect of these two agents may rarely occur in the tissues and fluids of the body, since the optimum proportions for synergy are probably not obtained except in the blood. Consequently, most of the activity of the combination is due to trimethoprim, and the fact that most skin rashes following co-trimoxazole are due to the sulphamethoxazole component has led to the suggestion that trimethoprim should be used alone in both urinary tract and chest infections.

Trimethoprim

Increasing use of trimethoprim has led, in some areas[8], to increasing resistance among common pathogens of both high-level chromosomal resistance and low-level resistance. High-level resistance is due to a transposon gene that may mobilize from the bacterial chromosome to a plasmid and so spread between strains of bacteria.

Tetracyclines and Chloramphenicol

Doxycycline

These antimicrobial agents have little role in elderly patients. Resistance to tetracyclines is common amongst streptococci, staphylococci and Gram-negative bacilli. Tetracyclines may lead to gastrointestinal irritation and superinfection with *Candida* spp. in the vagina, mouth and gut. These antibiotics increase amino-acid breakdown and consequently may worsen or precipitate renal dysfunction. Doxycycline, however, is free of this side-effect and is better absorbed from the intestinal tract than other tetracyclines.

Chloramphenicol

This can depress bone marrow function and, in a separate side-effect, may very rarely induce aplastic anaemia. It should be reserved for the specific indications of typhoid fever, meningitis and perhaps for clinically resistant chest infection.

Other Antibiotics in Current Use

Metronidazole

This is an efficient bactericidal agent restricted in its activity to obligate anaerobic bacteria, for which it is the antibacterial of choice. It is absorbed well from the gastrointestinal tract by either the oral or rectal route and penetrates body tissues efficiently. It is an important component of the antimicrobial treatment of abdominal infection of all kinds, as well as of pelvic infection in the female. It should also be used in treating lung abscess and empyema and infections of the soft tissues of the mouth and neck. It is particularly important in the treatment of brain abscess. Tinidazole is a similar agent which may be preferred to metronidazole in the treatment of *Giardia lamblia* infection and in amoebiasis, depending on further trials.

Vancomycin

This has become important in recent years in the treatment of pseudomembranous colitis where it is used in a dose of 125 or 250mg orally 6-hourly. It is also the treatment of choice for methicillin-resistant (that is flucloxacillin-resistant) *Staph. aureus* infections. The newer parenteral preparations of this agent appear to be less toxic than those of several years ago, but must still be administered intravenously. Ototoxicity and nephrotoxicity should be watched for, particularly if used with gentamicin.

Fucidin

This is a valuable antibiotic for serious and/or deep infections with *Staph. aureus*. It should always be used in combination with flucloxacillin or erythromycin since resistance to it may develop rapidly if used on its own. In order to preserve its efficacy for serious infection it should not be used topically, since surface application may lead to resistance by *Staph. aureus*.

FUTURE DEVELOPMENTS IN ANTIBIOTIC THERAPY

The large number of available antibiotics and the apparently endless development of new varieties may lead to a false sense of security. Many new antibiotics are a variation on a previous drug, often with improved properties but with a similar action on bacteria as their predecessors.

The development of drugs with better activity against fungi and a wider range of activity against viruses than those available is still needed.

Absorption from the Gastrointestinal Tract

The absorption of most antibacterials from the gut is poor, even for those forms of antibiotics specifically adapted for this route, such as flucloxacillin, amoxycillin and erythromycin stearate. Flucloxacillin was developed for better oral absorption from cloxacillin, and although the latter antibiotic is more active against *Staph. aureus* it has become common to use flucloxacillin by parenteral routes as well as the oral route. Prodrugs, where the antibiotic molecule is modified to allow better absorption and then converted to the original form by tissue enzymes in the gut wall, also improve absorption. Talampicillin and pondocillin are esters of ampicillin which, once absorbed, yield ampicillin and the ester side chain.

Better absorption of these antibiotics, and of doxycycline compared to other tetracyclines, reduces the side-effect of diarrhoea, but absorption still remains incomplete even with these modified forms and there is considerable room for improvement.

Ciprofloxacin

In this direction, the development of the substituted quinolones is significant. These compounds are related to nalidixic acid and cinoxacin which are already available, and perhaps the most promising of the new agents is ciprofloxacin [9]. This agent is sufficiently absorbed from the gut to provide adequate blood levels, in view of the very low inhibitory and bactericidal concentrations required. The broad spectrum of antibacterial activity, resistance to beta-lactamases, oral administration and high potency offer considerable promise.

Delivery to Site of Infection and Penetration of Bacteria

Once absorbed antibiotics are delivered to the site of infection by the bloodstream. Penetration of tissues and of areas of inflammation is dependent, in general, upon the diffusion gradient between the blood and different body compartments. More specific modes of delivery are possible. It has been suggested that liposomes could be constructed to contain antibiotics [10]. These might then be carried to sites of infection within polymorphs, and it is possible that some specificity for 'homing in' and concentrating at the site of infection might be provided by attaching antibodies to the liposome surface. It is also possible that antibiotics might be directly attached to immunoglobulins if the nature of the infecting organism is known so that susceptible bacteria might be captured in the immediate vicinity of the antibiotic.

Once the antibiotic is in the surrounding medium of the bacterium, it must penetrate the bacterial cell in order to reach target sites. The most effective resistance of bacteria to penicillins and cephalosporins is by the production of beta-lactamases, and many of these antibiotics are destroyed by the enzyme before bacterial penetration can occur. The development of beta-lactamase-resistant penicillins and cephalosporins and of the use of clavulanic acid partially overcome this problem, but there are still certain bacteria which produce beta-lactamases able to destroy the more recent cephalosporins and resist clavulanic acid. Only further experience will tell whether these strains of bacteria will become clinically important or can transfer the ability to produce these enzymes to other bacteria.

Further research is required into the mode of entry of antibiotics into bacteria, and it is possible that antibiotic molecules will be modified to improve bacterial penetration. Those antibiotics that are able to inhibit and kill pseudomonas strains are those that can enter the bacterial cell, since this organism resists antibiotics largely by their exclusion.

Once within the bacterial cell, antibiotics must then attach to their target sites. Penicillins and cephalosporins combine with enzymes or 'penicillin-binding proteins' which are involved in the construction of the bacterial cell wall. Different varieties of penicillins and cephalosporins bind to different enzymes, leading to different morphological effects on the bacterial cell. More detailed knowledge of the affinity of antibiotics to their targets may lead to more efficient antibiotics. This applies also to those antibiotics that attach to ribosomes or affect the bacterial cytoplasmic membrane.

Spectrum of Activity

When the infecting organism is known, it is preferable to use a narrow-spectrum agent effective against the pathogen but inactive against the normal bacterial flora and other potential pathogens of the body. This reduces the possibility of side-effects and of the selective pressure for bacterial resistance. When the pathogen has not been isolated, a broad spectrum of activity may well be necessary, although once the site of infection is known the range of organisms causing the infection can be narrowed. However, broad activity and the advantage of using a single agent instead of two or three has been the motive force for much research by the pharmaceutical industry. Consequently, agents with wide activity are still being produced and the cephalosporins are an example of excessive response to this perceived need. The cephalosporin spectrum is not complete and these antibacterials are inactive against many anaerobes and some coliforms as well as enterococci.

Thienamycin

A new modification of the penicillin molecule has been discovered which may rectify these deficiencies. Thienamycin [11] was discovered in cultures of *Streptomyces cattleya;* a modification of a side-chain produced N-formimidoyl thienamycin or imipenem which was stable in solution. Unfortunately, the compound is rapidly destroyed in the kidney by renal dipeptidase, but cilastatin inhibits this enzyme and by mixing it with imipenem activity of the latter is preserved. The combined agent is highly potent and has a wide spectrum of activity, including the enterococci and *Pseudomonas* spp., as well as a wide variety of anaerobes. The drug is given parenterally but future developments will be watched with interest.

Dosage Frequency and Duration of Treatment

Antibiotics with long half-lives can be given with reduced frequency. Some newer agents which have longer than usual half-lives in serum have been marketed for twice-daily or once-daily dosage, but prolonged intervals between doses with serum levels below inhibitory concentrations may be detrimental. It is true to say, however, that the pattern of dosage of antibiotics has developed incidentally or for historical reasons. Evidence is needed to know whether high doses can be given at infrequent intervals or whether it is better to use lower doses at frequent intervals. Similarly, it is not known whether a continuous infusion of antibiotic giving a steady serum level at an effective concentration would be more efficient than intermittent doses. There is some evidence that in neutropenic patients a constant infusion may be marginally more effective than intermittent doses, and with the advent of reliable syringe pumps and convenient peripheral venous catheters this mode of therapy may become more common.

Similarly, the optimum duration of dosage is uncertain; it is usually suggested that parenteral administration continues for 1 or 2 days after the temperature has returned to normal. It is probable that most of the infecting organisms are killed by the initial doses of antibiotic, if these are adequate and can reach the site of infection. One study, from an area in Africa where meningitis is seasonal, has revealed that meningococcal meningitis is cured in the majority of patients by a single dose of benzylpenicillin. Further studies in this direction both in animal models of infection and in patients are justified.

Antibiotic Policies and Education

The multiplicity of antibiotics and their safety for the patient has led to a low threshold of use. There is now much evidence to show that high usage of antibiotics is associated with increasing bacterial resistance and that reduction in use is followed by reduced resistance. Many doctors now feel that a free-for-all approach to antibiotic prescribing is outdated and that some form of antibiotic policy would be acceptable to them. Antibiotic policies perform several functions; they can formalize optimal use of antibiotics in areas such as surgical prophylaxis and chest infection, and restrict topical use. They may suggest appropriate antibiotics for certain infections and by adopting an agreed formulary restrict the number of antibiotics available to prescribers. The latter policy may reduce costs, and allows a change in the recommended drugs if and when increasing resistance by bacteria occurs. In order to preserve the antibiotics already available, a much-needed future development is increasing education and vigilance about their use.

BACTERIOLOGICAL DIAGNOSIS

Blood Culture

Blood culture is a relatively cheap bacteriological investigation and should be taken before antibiotics are started in any elderly patient with pyrexia [12]. Blood culture is a valuable investigation in any age group where infection may be present. The clinical presentation of septicaemia in older patients may be without clinical signs other than confusion, and blood cultures should be taken routinely from all confused elderly patients. In infections in the chest it is frequently found that the organism can be cultured from blood but not from sputum taken at the same time, and in my experience this is specially so with *Streptococcus pneumoniae* where a lobar consolidation may prevent sputum formation.

Sputum Examination

Sputum is a highly unreliable bacteriological specimen. The reasons for this are several fold; the exudate from an area of pneumonitis or consolidation in the lung must travel the length of the airways and through the mouth before expectoration, and will always be contaminated by the abundant normal flora of the mouth. The contaminating normal flora may overgrow the pathogen on culture plates. On the other hand, a few patients are carriers of *Strep. pneumoniae* and/or *H. influenzae,* and isolation from sputum of these organisms may not be relevant to the infection in the lung. Sputum is an unhomogeneous substance and purulent lung exudate may be mixed with saliva and mucus, which will dilute any pathogens present. The small portion taken for culture may not be representative of the lung secretions. Perhaps only one in 10 or one in 20 sputum samples yields a result of value to the clinician. There is a strong case for more invasive procedures such as transtracheal aspiration and needle aspiration of lung tissue. The latter procedure can often be undertaken by radiologists under X-ray guidance. The amount of tissue retrieved is sufficient for histology as well as bacterial culture and Gram film (provided it is not formalinized!). Both of these procedures are less invasive than open lung biopsy which is a procedure of last resort.

Urine Examination

The examination of urine is less reliable than it may appear; it is difficult to obtain a true midstream specimen from a bed-bound immobile patient and samples for culture tend to be taken from urine collected in bedpans or urinals. Inevitably, the organisms so obtained originate from the utensil rather than the patient, or from both. In patients who are catheterized the urine sample should be obtained by syringe and needle from the catheter lumen, as close as possible to the urethral opening. Specimens obtained from the urine reservoir bag are more likely to grow contaminating organisms from the stored urine or from the hands involved in manipulating the reservoir outlet. In the normal, but infirm, female elderly patient the urine stream is easily contaminated from the labia or nearby skin.

These problems should be borne in mind when assessing urine culture reports. Although pyuria is not a necessary accompaniment of urinary infection, it may be wise to repeat urine cultures if pyuria is absent or there were difficulties in collecting the specimen.

Patients who are permanently catheterized will inevitably have infected urine. Usually several organisms are present in a mixed infection and the usual recommendation is to treat only if symptoms of upper renal tract infection are present. Suprapubic aspiration yields a reliable specimen and should, preferably, be more widely practised.

When a urine sample yields a mixed growth in the presence of pyuria, the test should be repeated with precautions against contamination. If mixed organisms are consistently obtained from reliable specimens it may be necessary to treat with a broad-spectrum first-line agent, such as co-trimoxazole, provided symptoms are present, and then repeat cultures after treatment. When there is evidence of pyelonephritis blood cultures will be valuable.

Pus or Tissue Specimens

In soft tissue, bone and abdominal infections, pus or tissue are more reliable specimens for bacteriology than swabs. Swabs tend to dry out unless sent in transport medium, and they are inefficient, being poor both at picking up bacteria and releasing bacteria onto the culture plate. Even a small quantity of pus in the barrel of a syringe, which can be sent to the laboratory in a plastic specimen bag, is worthwhile.

Stool Examination

Stool examination now yields more pathogens than ever before. Salmonella, shigella and campylobacter are easy to culture, while rotavirus and *Clostridium difficile* and its toxin can now be sought routinely.

Needle Aspiration

In suspected osteomyelitis, liver abscess and abdominal abscess a radiologist may be able to needle aspirate from the suspected site of infection, and this may reveal the causative organisms without the necessity for operation – sometimes an advantage in a frail, very elderly patient, who may respond to antibiotic treatment alone.

Bacteriology Request Forms

It is a homily, but a true one, that the more information given on a bacteriology request form the better will be the result. If antibiotics, for instance, have already been given to the patient, this should be declared since it may be possible to neutralize penicillin-type drugs and to inactivate or dilute other antibiotics. Information of the site of infection will help the bacteriologist determine the nature of the organism isolated and information of a recent operation may forewarn of a cross-infection hazard. Operation wounds should be distinguished from pressure ulcers or stasis ulcers, since the clinical relevance of different bacteria will vary between the two types of lesion.

New Techniques

New techniques of diagnosis include serological and biochemical methods of detecting bacterial antigens in body tissues. Their advantage is sensitivity, rapidity and the ability to detect breakdown products or dead bacteria, as well as live bacteria as required by traditional cultural methods.

Latex particles coated with appropriate antibody will agglutinate in the presence of antigen, and this technique is now used to diagnose the common types of bacterial meningitis. Serological methods, such as enzyme-linked immunosorbent assay (ELISA) are available to detect rotavirus in stool, as well as antibodies to hepatitis A and B. Many laboratories have automated blood culture procedures by using radioactive nutrients in the media; bacteria metabolize these to radioactive CO_2 which is detected in the head space of the blood culture bottles. Positive cultures are then further categorized by traditional means. Gas liquid chromatography is potentially able to 'finger print' bacteria by their metabolites, and Coulter counters could become adapted to enumerating bacteria and cells in urine specimens.

However, both mechanization and automation are in their infancy in microbiology, and labour-intensive manual bench work will remain the chief approach to diagnosis for several, perhaps many, years.

References

1. Moss, F., McNicol, M. W., McSwiggan, D. A. and Miller, D. L. (1981). Survey of antibiotic prescribing in a district general hospital. *Lancet*, **2**, 349–52
2. Ball, P., Banford, T., Gilbert, J., Johnson, T. and Mitchard, M. (1978). Prolonged serum elimination half-life of amoxycillin in the elderly. *J. Antimicrob. Chemother.*, **4**, 385
3. Humber, M. W., Eykyn, S. J. and Phillips, I. (1980). Staphylococcal bacteraemia, fusidic acid and jaundice. *Br. Med. J.* **2**, 1495–8
4. Leading article (1983). Antimicrobials and haemastasis, *Lancet*, **1**, 510–11
5. Lipsky, J. J. (1983). N-methyl-thio-tetrazole inhibition of the gamma carboxylation of glutamic acid: possible mechanism for antibiotic associated hypoprothrombinaemia. *Lancet* **2**, 192–3
6. Bennett, W. M., Singer I. and Coggins, C. M. (1970). A practical guide to drug usage in adult patients with impaired renal function. *J. Am. Med. Assoc.*, **214**, 1468
7. Sharpstone, P. (1977). Diseases of the urinary system. Prescribing for patients with renal failure. *Br. Med. J.* **2**, 36
8. Towner, K. J. and Wise, P. J. (1983). Transferable resistance plasmids as a contributory cause of increasing trimethoprim resistance in general practice. *J. Antimicrob. Chemother.* **11**, 33–9
9. Reeves, D. S. (ed.) (1984). Current topic: ciprofloxacin: microbiology and pharmacology. *Eur. J. Clin. Microbiol.* **3**, 325–75
10. Fendler, J. H. and Romero, A. (1977). Liposomes as drug carriers. *Life Sci.*, **20**, 1109
11. Wise, R., Andrews, J. M. and Patel, N. (1981). N-formimidoyl thienamycin a novel β-lactam: an *in vitro* comparison with other β-lactam antibiotics. *J. Antimicrob. Chemother.*, **7**, 521–529
12. Denham, M. J. and Goodwin, G. S. (1977). The value of blood cultures in geriatric practice. *Age Ageing*, **6**, 85

General Reading

Garrod, L. P., Lambert, H. P. and O'Grady, F. (1981). *Antibiotic and Chemotherapy*. (Edinburgh: Churchill Livingstone)

Geddes, A. M., Levy, S. B., Wise, R., Ball, A. P., Neu, H. C., Phillips, I., Reeves, D. S., Kucers, A., Bartlett, J. G. and Cohen, J. (1982). *Good Antimicrobial Prescribing: A Lancet Review*. (London: *Lancet*)

Tyrell, D. A. J., Phillips, I., Goodwin, C. S. and Blowers, R. (1979). *Microbial Disease: The Use of the Laboratory in Diagnosis, Treatment and Control*. (London: Edward Arnold)

Selwyn, S. (1980). *The Beta-lactam Antibiotics: Penicillins and Cephalosporins in Perspective*. (London: Hodder and Stoughton)

2

Infection and Immunity in Old Age

R. A. FOX

INTRODUCTION

The human body protects itself from infection in a number of ways (Table 2.1), and these protective mechanisms become less efficient with advancing age. The relative importance of the different forms of defence are not clear, and it may be that natural barriers to infection are of greater significance than acquired immunity. Nevertheless waning immunity appears to be directly correlated with the rising incidence of infection. Although many diseases such as cerebrovascular disease become increasingly common in old age, they are not thought to be directly linked to deteriorating immunity. The evidence for the link between infection and impaired immunity in old age is circumstantial, but the role of immunity in infection is so important and well studied that it appears safe to conclude that waning immunity directly contributes to the significant morbidity and mortality from infection in old age. To understand the link we need to understand the nature of the immune response.

Table 2.1 Defence against infection

Natural barriers	Non-immunological	Immunological
Intact skin or mucosa	polymorphonuclear phagocytes	humoral (antibodies)
Hygiene	opsonins	
Cleaning	complement	cell-mediated
Motility	acute phase proteins	(cells)
Secretions		

23

NATURAL BARRIERS TO INFECTION

The body has considerable natural resistance to micro-organisms. The skin is impermeable to most infectious agents and provides an important line of defence. The natural secretions produced by the skin and attached organs, such as sweat and sebum, provide a hostile microenvironment for most bacteria. The continuous shedding of the skin by wear and tear with replenishment also ensures a degree of cleanliness.

The same is true of the other surfaces which interface with the outside world. The mucosal surface of the gastrointestinal tract provides an effective barrier against infection. The integrity of the mucosal lining is of paramount importance and this is protected by a layer of mucus which blocks the attachment of micro-organisms. Within the mucus are several antibacterial agents like secretory IgA which is discussed below. The surface is continually cleaned by the passage of material through the gut. The only sites where bacteria abound are where there is considerable stasis such as the colon. Motility is thus an important factor in defence. Access to the gastrointestinal tract is impeded by the performance of simple hygienic measures and by the barrier of gastric acid.

Similar strategies for defence exist with the other mucosal surfaces such as the genitourinary tract. Various factors including the rapid flow of urine serve to prevent adherence and reduce the risk of infection or permanent colonization.

The factors which are present in secretions which act as barriers to infection include muramidase in saliva and tears, spermine in prostatic secretions, zinc and iron-containing proteins in the genital tract and acid in the stomach. Various factors in the serum also play an important role in defence, and these are termed acute phase proteins. C-reactive protein, serum amyloid A and the various complement components are examples of these. The exact role of all these factors is not fully understood. However, it appears that some of the complement components play a major role in defence together with the phagocytic cells by acting as opsonins. Opsonization of bacteria renders them more attractive to the phagocyte and thus promotes phagocytosis.

The polymorphonuclear leukocyte plays a major role in defence, although it is, in the strict sense, non-immunological. Tissue invasion, damage and immunological reactions all act to release chemotactic factors. Neutrophils migrate along the chemotactic gradient to the site of invasion and there phagocytoze opsonized particles. The polymorphonuclear leukocyte contains many microbicidal activities effective against micro-organisms. Intraleukocyte killing involves the generation of oxidizing agents as hydrogen peroxide, the generation of halides such as chloride ion and the generation of singlet oxygen.

The exact roles of these non-specific activities vary with the infection. In certain situations, such as invasion with *Staphylococcus aureus,* the polymorphonuclear leukocyte appears to be the most important.

The other phagocytic cells are those of the monocyte/macrophage series. These cells have a variety of functions, including very important roles in the early stages of the immune response; however, they are also wandering scavengers and internalize macromolecules, particles and organisms by phagocytosis and pinocytosis. Phagocytosis is enhanced by opsonization. These cells are particularly important in defence against agents like viruses and fungi. Interaction with the micro-organisms or their components such as endotoxin results in activation of the macrophage. In this state the cell can release enzymes and becomes cytocidal, killing organisms and cells such as tumour cells. In this state the monocyte is much more efficient at phagocytosis and killing.

THE IMMUNE RESPONSE

Background

It has been known for many years that individuals who recover from an infectious illness are usually protected from subsequent attack. The study of this phenomenon led to the discovery of the science of immunology. Soluble molecules or cells are capable of inducing an immune response, and they are known as immunogens. They contain on their surfaces molecular configurations which are known as antigenic determinants. Immunogenic particles are taken up by cells of the monocyte/macrophage series, and the antigenic determinants then presented to the lymphocytes to induce an immune response. The immune response takes place in the lymph node which drains the tissue which is the site of microbiological invasion, or within the bloodstream. The primed macrophage interacts with the lymphocytes.

Lymphocytes are produced in the bone marrow and migrate to the bloodstream where they circulate, some leaving to populate lymph nodes, the spleen and the various tissues. The lymphocytes fall into two main categories: those that mature by passage through the bursa of Fabricius in birds or its equivalent in man (which is thought to be gut-associated lymph tissue) the B lymphocyte; and those that mature by passage through the thymus, the T lymphocyte. These cells are responsible for the products of the immune response, namely the antibodies from the B cells and the sensitized T lymphocytes (Figure 2.1).

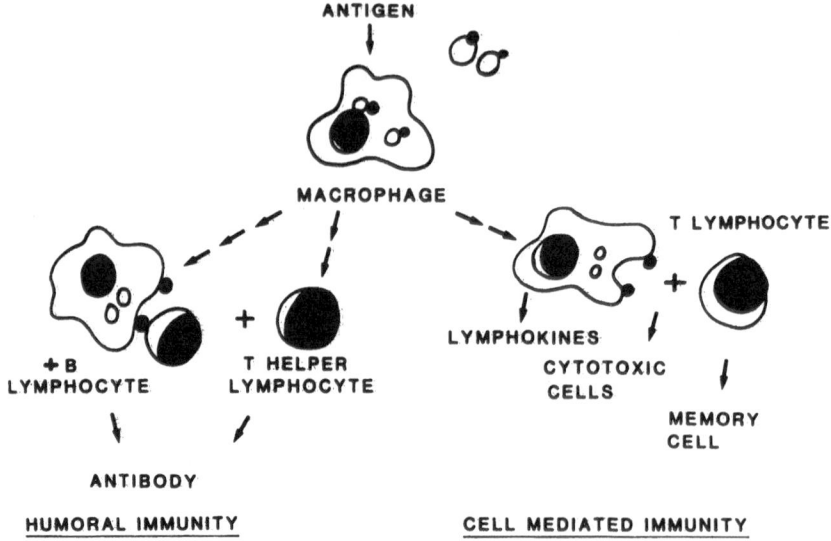

Figure 2.1 The immune response

Humoral Immunity

The primed macrophage reacts with the B lymphocyte, and the B cell is transformed. The result of this transformation is the production of increased numbers of cells and the release of antibodies. Antibodies are serum proteins which belong to one of five major immunoglobulin classes. This sequence of events from initial antigen recognition to the production of immunoglobulin and subsequent interaction with antigen is referred to as humoral immunity. For some antigens the above sequence of events is correct but for others the B lymphocyte needs to be helped by cells from the T lymphocyte series – T helper cells. This subpopulation is discussed in the next section. The net result of such help is the production of antibodies.

The five classes of immunoglobulins are A, D, E, G and M. Each molecule consists of two heavy chains which determine the type and the properties of the different immunoglobulins. IgM is a large molecule which is found only within the intravascular compartment; it forms the first antibodies in the immune response and is efficient at agglutinating foreign particles, and at activating complement. IgG is present in high concentration in the serum, and is produced in sequence to the IgM production in the primary antibody response, and is the main component of the secondary antibody response. IgA is also found in the serum but its main role is as secretory IgA, being locally produced in the mucosa in various parts of the body such as the respiratory and gastrointestinal tracts. This molecule does not activate complement, but is effective in agglutinating particles which are then cleared more easily. The function of IgD is not clear, and it is found mainly in the serum. IgE binds to mast cells and plays the major role in immediate hypersensitivity reactions.

The importance of humoral immunity in any particular immune reaction appears to be determined by the invading micro-organism. For example, in the case of *Streptococcus pneumoniae* humoral immunity seems to be the most important, and antibody-producing cells can be found within 48 hours of experimental inoculation. In this situation the major role of the antibodies is in opsonization which overcomes the antiphagocytic effect of the pneumococcal capsule.

Cell-mediated Immunity

The primed macrophage interacts with the T lymphocyte with the result that there is clonal expansion of the T lymphocytes. These cells are capable of binding the sensitizing antigen (immunogen) which may then be destroyed since the T cell can become cytocidal. The sensitized, transforming T cell also produces various biologically active molecules which stimulate other cells and whose net effect is to augment the immune response. These molecules are known as lymphokines, and examples include interferon (active against viral infections), macrophage activation factor which promotes the increased activity of macrophages (discussed above), interleukin 1 which has many effects including the production of fever and the synthesis of acute phase proteins, and interleukin 2 which recruits other T lymphocytes and supports proliferation. Some of the sensitized cells are very long-living and circulate within the bloodstream and the lymphatics as memory cells, conferring immunity.

Cell-mediated immunity is detected by the presence of circulating sensitized cells by means of skin testing – the classical delayed hypersensitivity reaction. This form of immunity is particularly important in defence against infections like tuberculosis and varicella zoster. It is the type of immunity involved in protection against cancer and transplants.

The T lymphocyte is also responsible for controlling or modulating functions. The T cells can be identified as distinct subgroups, by the presence of specific membrane antigens. All T lymphocytes are detected by monoclonal antibody to a surface antigen referred to as T3+. The subpopulation which stains for T8+ has suppressor or cytotoxic characteristics. It has been found that if increased numbers of these cells are added to an *in vitro* immune response, that response is suppressed. These cells are either non-specific and suppress all immune reactions or are specific to the antigen. The other subgroup of T cells is the helper T lymphocyte which stains for T4+. These are the cells which co-operate with B cells and provide soluble factors that amplify the response.

These two types of cells seem to be important in all immune responses and serve a modulator role that adjusts the level of the immune response, to 'set the level of the thermostat'. Naturally there are other controlling mechanisms and the immune reactions are exceedingly complex, but for the purpose of this discussion they do not need to be explored.

AGEING AND THE IMMUNE RESPONSE

Non-Immunological Mechanisms

Ageing produces changes in all tissues, and it is obvious that there is change within the skin and the mucosal surfaces throughout the body. These changes are likely to contribute to the changing pattern of infection encountered in old age, but have been little studied. The observation that the rate of oropharyngeal colonization increases in old age and with increasing degrees of dependency[1] suggests change. The frequency with which bacteria adhere to the epithelial cells of the genitourinary tract increases with advancing age, and this would suggest some change in the characteristics of the cells. This certainly appears to be an area that is worthy of exploration (Table 2.2).

Table 2.2 Ageing and defence

Natural barrier	Non-immunological	Immunological
Increased adherence of microbes	impaired recruitment of polymorphs	impaired antibody response
Reduced gastric acidity		increased autoantibodies
Reduced mucus production		impaired T cell function (helper and suppressor)

Other natural barriers to infection become less efficient with age, and a good example would be the acid within the stomach. Achlorhydria becomes increasingly common in old age, being found in about one-third of those over 60. Lack of acid has been known to be important in various enteric infections including cholera and shigella. A recent report from a geriatric unit found that all patients who developed shigella infection had low acid production due to the presence of associated disease such as pernicious anaemia or the administration of antacids, including H_2 blocking agents[2]. This emphasizes that in this age group one needs to be thinking of disease and pharmacological agents as well as the process of ageing itself.

Complement levels and opsonic activity have been measured and not found to deteriorate with age. The situation with regard to the phagocytic cells is less clear although my conclusion is that there is little change due to age itself. We have found that in healthy elderly subjects chemilumines-cence[3] and nitroblue tetrazolium (NBT) reduction[4], both of which measure the respiratory burst of polymorphs, do not change with age. There is evidence, however, that these functions are adversely affected by many of the diseases that are common in this age group such as cancer and uraemia. Phagocytosis also appears to be unaffected by ageing[5]. There are isolated reports of impaired chemiluminescence or adherence in old age but these are not consistent. I conclude that the non-specific response of polymor-phonuclear leukocytes remains intact in old age. However there does appear to be a problem with the production or release of these cells (recruitment), since the finding of a normal white blood cell count in the presence of infection is not uncommon in old age. In fact this appears to become increasingly more common with advancing age, at least with pneumococcal bacteraemia[6]. In our studies we found a number of people with proven infection, a positive NBT test indicating the presence of activated polymorphs and a normal white blood cell count. Thus the cells respond normally with a respiratory burst but there is no increase in numbers. This area needs further study.

In the context of an inflammatory response and their phagocytic capacity, the cells of the monocyte/macrophage series appear to function normally. Macrophages from aged hosts phagocytoze and kill normally. In fact the cells from old animals appear to be activated and to have 'supernormal' phagocytosis. This phenomenon is thought to lead to impairment of some of the other functions since phagocytozed particles and their antigens are digested more rapidly in these circumstances. In this case the antigens will not be expressed on the cell surfaces and an immune response will not be mounted. It is also suggested that this increased phagocytosis of the acti-vated macrophage contributes to the rising incidence of cancer in old age[7]. It is postulated that since tumour antigens are weak antigens they are more rapidly destroyed, thus making an immune response less likely.

Humoral Immunity

The number of circulating lymphocytes does not appear to change consis-tently with advancing age. The stem cells which give rise to these cells do not undergo significant change with age, although in some species of experimen-tal animal the number of cells that are capable of colonizing the spleen do decrease in old age. The circulating B cells bearing immunoglobulin surface markers remain constant with advancing age but the number of colony-forming units decreases[7]. The B cells undergo some qualitative changes like a reduction in the density of surface immunoglobulin and the presence of altered mitochondria.

Some of the clinical observations, like the rising incidence of monoclonal gammopathies, suggest that there might be significant changes in B cell function, more than can be accounted for by minor qualitative changes so far discussed. In experimental animals antigen-induced primary antibody responses decline with age, but secondary antibody responses remain unaffected[8]. The results in man are somewhat conflicting but in general show that the response to bacterial and viral vaccines does not decline with age[9]. More recent studies with influenza and pneumococcal vaccines suggest that these vaccines retain their efficacy in old age but that the maximum response is lower and delayed and the drop off sooner [10]. It is likely that the antibody produced is of inferior quality; at least in experimental animals the avidity declines[11].

The humoral immune responses that decline would appear to be those which can be designated T-dependent, and for this reason the explanation put forward is that any change detected is secondary to thymic involution and the decline in T cell function.

Cell-mediated Immunity

The thymus gland which plays a central role in the maturation of T lymphocytes undergoes marked involutional change from puberty onwards. Thymic involution has been a central theme in the description of changes in the immune response with advancing age. The involution of the thymus seems to be reflected in the function of the T cells, although there is no change in the numbers of circulating T lymphocytes. *In vitro* proliferation in response to certain stimulants such as the plant mitogens phytohaemagglutinin and concanavalin A deteriorates with advancing age, although this change has not been found by all observers. More recent work has focused on the various cellular interactions and it has been shown that with ageing there is deterioration in different parts of the immune response. The primed and activated macrophage releases a chemical messenger, namely interleukin 1 (IL–1), which stimulates the T lymphocyte. In experimental animals ageing appears to have an adverse effect on the production of IL–1, but this has not been confirmed in man. However this substance is worthy of further study because of the many other effects that it has including stimulation of the hypothalamus to produce fever in response to infection. The T lymphocytes which are transformed then produce many other lymphokines including IL–2 which supports the further proliferation of T cells. IL–2 production has been shown to be impaired in old age in both experimental animals and man.

In man there appears to be an increasing chance of negative delayed hypersensitivity skin tests with advancing age. This is true for both previously established immunity and for new contact with contact sensitizers like dinitrochlorobenzene (DNCB). It is of interest that one of these studies revealed that those patients with impaired delayed hypersensitivity (anergy) were more likely to die within the next 2 years than those patients with intact responses[12].

The overall change in function appears to be a general decline, greater than can be explained by the minor qualitative changes observed within these cells, and certainly not accounted for by any change in numbers. The explanation appears to rest with the thymic involution, in that the T lymphocytes are unable to mature normally and become functionally deficient. The effects on the T cell are also reflected in some of the changes that are seen within the subpopulations of T cells.

If the age changes are due to the thymic deficiency then replacement with young thymus or with thymic extract should correct the deficiency. Recent work indicates that there is some restoration of function if fetal thymus is transplanted into old mice, or if thymic hormone is injected. However, much more work needs to be done before this can be considered a possible treatment modality in man.

Autoimmunity and the Role of Modulator Cells

The subpopulations of T lymphocytes that subserve a modulating or controlling function undergo some changes with advancing age. The absolute numbers of suppressor T cells as measured by monoclonal antibody to T8+ appear to decline with advancing age[13] and T helper cells remain constant (T4+). Earlier studies were less clear cut, but the results of studies into functional aspects help to clarify the issue. T helper function as measured by ability to help in response to tetanus vaccination declines with ageing[14]. T suppressor function may also decline in man, although in some experimental animals there is an increase[9].

The evidence that has accumulated leads to the conclusion that there is a loss of suppressor cells that control autoantibody production with advancing age. The result of this is that there is an increased incidence of autoantibodies in old age. The autoantibodies are usually in low titre. Those most frequently found are to nuclear, gastric parietal cell and thyroid antigens. They have not been directly implicated in the pathogenesis of disease.

As there is a decline in the production of antibodies to extrinsic antigens, there is an increased propensity to produce antibodies to intrinsic or self-antigens. These changes are related to the changes in the T cell populations and most authorities relate this to thymic involution. It has been pointed out that there needs to be a stimulus to fire off the B cells to produce the autoantibodies in the first place which the defective T cells then fail to suppress. Polyclonal activators like endotoxin might be responsible[15]. A recent hypothesis postulates that the accumulation of circulating endotoxins due to altered colonic function and deteriorating Kupffer cell function produces these changes and in fact are the major age changes of importance in relation to immune function[16]. In other words the changes in immune function that we have discussed are secondary to environmental factors (Figure 2.2).

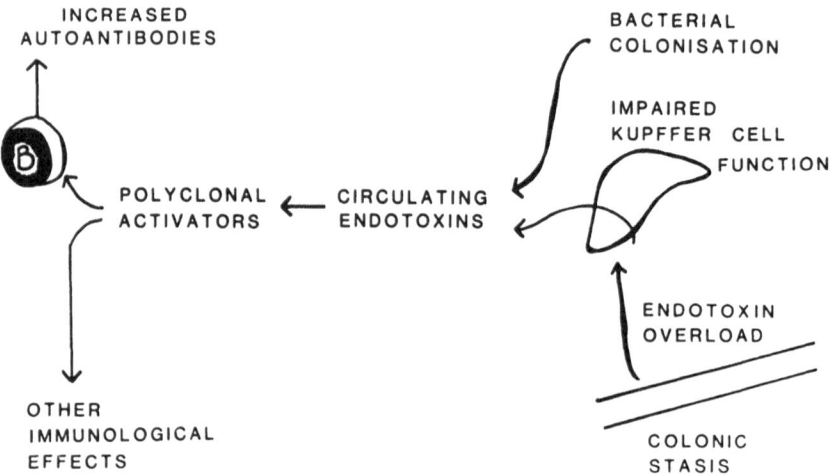

Figure 2.2 Endotoxin and autoantibody production

WANING IMMUNITY AND INFECTIONS

Role of Impaired Immunity

Ageing is not the only factor in the older patient that contributes to impaired immunity. We have seen that mobility influences colonization, which in turn may influence the immune response. There is a great deal of evidence that many of the diseases that are common in old age are associated with impaired immune responsiveness, for example cancer, leukaemia, uraemia or liver disease. A problem with some of the earlier studies of aged populations was that these factors were not carefully controlled for and thus the impaired immunity attributed to ageing may have been more related to the diseases. A recent study helps to clarify this issue, in that malnutrition, which is known to impair immune responsiveness, was found to be common in a group of elderly subjects studied. When the malnutrition was partially corrected with supplements there was very significant improvement in the immunological tests such as *in vitro* lymphocyte transformation[17]. However the deficiencies were not completely corrected.

Older patients are therefore likely to be immunodeficient, to a variable degree, either due to the ageing process or to associated disease. Does this immunodeficiency directly contribute to the prevalence of infection? The direct evidence is limited. Patients who were found to be anergic by skin testing were found to have a significantly higher death rate over the next 2 years after testing[12]. This is of great interest but the mode of death in the anergic patients was not made clear. Patients who have recurrent or continuous bacteriuria are more likely to die[18], but we know nothing of their immunological responsiveness.

Individuals who succumb to varicella zoster infection in old age, when compared to those individuals who do not, demonstrate lower levels of *in vitro* lymphocyte transformation. Here we have impaired immunity of a specific type linked with one infection. A recent study indicates that patients admitted to an acute hospital with pneumonia are more likely to die if they prove to be anergic to a battery of skin tests (Marrie, personal communication). It seems safe to conclude that immunodeficiency in old age is one of the important contributing factors to the increased infection rate in the elderly. Closely linked to the waning immunity is the reduced inflammatory response, and the importance of this in the clinical presentation of infection will become apparent in a subsequent section.

The Frequency of Infections

There is a great deal of data to confirm that not only does the frequency of infections increase with advancing age, but also the morbidity and mortality rates associated with infections increase. This observation holds true for infections of many different types and in different systems. The information found in other parts of this book clarifies this statement.

For example, infection of the urinary tract is an exceedingly common problem in old age. Bacteriuria is more common in females than males, and approximately 20% of the population over 65 have significant bacteriuria at any one time. In a proportion of the population this persists; in fact 10% of the total population over 55 are never free of infection. As disease and dependency increase the incidence of bacteriuria and symptomatic infection increases, so that the incidence reaches about 50% in a long-term care geriatric hospital.

We know that the risk of infection for old people entering hospital or nursing home is increased by two to five times compared with younger people[19]. Ageing itself appears to be a risk factor for the reasons already discussed. Resistance is also lowered by the presence of underlying diseases like leukaemia, lymphoma or diabetes. Concurrent therapy with antibiotics, corticosteroids or cytotoxic drugs will also lower resistance and increase the risk of infection. Procedures that are carried out on these patients are likely to increase the frequency of infection – for example catheterization of the bladder or intravenous catheterization.

The environment contributes to the high incidence, for example, the acute hospital with the different patients and their infections. In the long-term setting the elderly are in close confinement and therefore increasingly exposed not only to other residents but also to the staff. Outbreaks of tuberculosis and infective diarrhoea are well documented in this setting. The use of antibiotics in institutions contributes to the development of resistant strains of micro-organisms. The elderly themselves bring in fresh populations of microbes, for example the increased rate of oropharyngeal colonization is well documented. Oropharyngeal colonization in such a patient with limited mechanisms for clearing any aspirated organisms, reduced mobility and other associated diseases represents a typical scenario, illustrating the multiple contributions to the high rate of infection.

The high rate is applicable to most infections, and this is not due to a single deficit since defence will depend upon a variety of mechanisms. The phagocytic system, cellullar and humoral immunity are important to varying extents in the different types of infection. All are likely to be impaired to a greater or lesser extent in the older patient due to the effects of ageing or of disease itself.

Clinical Response

We have seen that the immune response tends to wane in old age, accompanied by a weakening of the inflammatory response. Examples of this have already been cited. There are many other changes that occur with advancing age, like the decrease in the ability to sense visceral pain. Many of the mechanisms which maintain homeostasis, and which are therefore very complex, also deteriorate with advancing age. The net result of these many changes is that in old age the symptoms and signs of disease become less florid and less clear cut. Infection may therefore become quite advanced before it manifests itself.

In the setting of old age the individual may have coexistent deterioration with impairment of function in many organs. This means that under normal or optimal environmental circumstances function may be adequate but there is minimal or no reserve. The individual may be living at home either independently or in a state of minimal dependence. However, if infection strikes additional stresses are placed upon the individual and the various systems within the body. With no reserve there is the potential for decompensation in many systems. The patient may then become confused, incontinent of urine and immobile in a very short period of time. The patient has what might be described as a geriatric presentation with the features of dependency and any of the so-called geriatric giants already mentioned (Figure 2.3).

This kind of geriatric presentation is more likely in the setting of increased

INFECTION

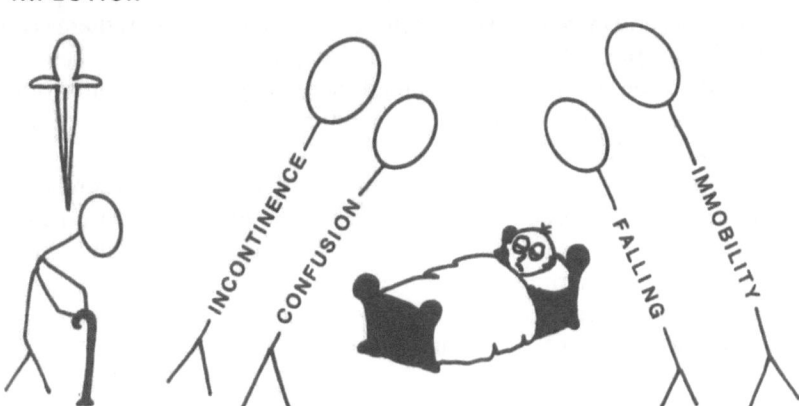

Figure 2.3 The 'geriatric giants' in the presentation of infection

dependency, but does occur in the very old who are living quite independently and were previously apparently well. This kind of presentation is more likely with advancing age, but it should be remembered that the majority of infections in the elderly present as they would at any other age with the typical signs and symptoms. The major differences would be that there is an increased likelihood of associated disease and recovery is likely to take longer.

The Importance of Diagnosis

The importance of early diagnosis needs to be stressed, since this will provide the best chance of successful treatment. This in turn provides the best opportunity for the patient to return to the previous level of independence. Treatment of an infection may allow successful management of multiple problems due to decompensation in multiple systems, for example, the control of incontinence, the return to mobility and the loss of confusion with return to mental clarity and competence.

Accurate diagnosis is made more likely by the taking of a careful history and a detailed physical examination. The body temperature needs to be recorded and should be taken accurately – the rectal route is preferred. The minimum investigations should include a complete blood count, with a statement on the smear and report on the presence of immature neutrophils, a chest radiograph and analysis of urine with culture. It is also desirable to have blood for measurement of electrolytes, sugar and liver function tests. The information from these tests will provide valuable clues as to the nature of the patient's underlying and complicating problems. At the very least there should be enough information available in order to identify the problem of infection, and in many instances the site of that infection. If there is no obvious site, but the nature of findings clearly point to infection then the patient needs to be carefully re-examined. Screening for infection should include vaginal examination in females, culture of urine and blood, and tuberculin skin testing.

Once the pathophysiological state is defined with a clear indication of the site of infection there needs to be an earnest attempt to obtain positive microbiological specimens. In this way the most appropriate therapy can be instituted. This is of paramount importance since it may be necessary to use very powerful antibiotics. Rapid, specific and effective treatment is the best way of limiting the risk of iatrogenic disease.

PREVENTION

Background

With advancing age death becomes more likely, and an important cause of death is infection. There would appear to be two major categories of infection. First, those that are inevitable concomitants of the dying process, and second, those that occur in a relatively healthy host and contribute to the death. Bronchopneumonia is found so commonly in those dying in hospital when they come to autopsy that in many cases it must be considered an untreatable concomitant. It is my experience that in certain patients, for example those dying within a long-term care ward with end-stage dementia and its sequelae of double incontinence and immobility, pneumonia is a different entity to that occurring in a young or old, healthy host. In this setting it is frequently unresponsive to antibiotics, and often the important determining factor with regard to recovery seems to be if the patient can be mobilized again. The challenge is to recognize these patients and allow them to die with dignity. The second group where there is infection contributing to death needs to be identified and treated. Death may be averted. It is also important to be able to recognize those at risk and hopefully to prevent the onset of infection. Prevention or, failing that, early effective therapy should be the aim and would contribute to a reduction in both morbidity and mortality among the elderly. Our study of autopsies revealed that there were significant numbers of patients dying in hospital where the diagnosis of infection was not considered during life[20].

There are specific approaches to the prevention of infection by means of immunization. There are also other approaches which are of equal if not greater importance. For example, the elderly frequently find themselves in situations of increased exposure to infection, from day care programmes and acute care hospitals to nursing homes and long-stay hospitals. Staff working within these institutions must be aware of the potential risks and should absent themselves at the first sign of infection. An outbreak of shigella dysentery that we studied appeared to have started among the patients through a member of the nursing staff. Other common examples, of course, are influenza and other respiratory infections.

A significant proportion of the ill elderly have confusion as a complicating problem, and with this comes an increased risk of poor hygiene. This must be remembered and great attention paid to hygienic practices. The high rate of nosocomial infection is partially the result of poor hygiene, for example the doctor's failure to wash his hands between seeing patients. Patients sharing a room with another patient with a urinary tract infection are much more likely to be infected, the common mode of transmission being hand carriage of the organisms. If outbreaks of infection do occur they should rapidly be contained by the most appropriate methods of isolation. This is a great challenge in the setting of a long-term care ward with a large number of demented patients. All elderly individuals need regular medical evaluation to determine that they are in optimal health and that there are no untreated problems. This is of great importance within the institutions and all problems should be managed as optimally as is possible. Furthermore, all unnecessary drugs should be discontinued and the state of nutrition assessed and if necessary optimized.

These factors should be taken into account in any caring situation, not just for the elderly. Older patients are undoubtedly more vulnerable but recognition that we are dealing with a population at increased risk means that we should take a hard look at immunization practices in general.

Efficacy of Immunization

Evidence has been presented that the primary antibody response is reduced as a result of ageing. Does this impairment represent a meaningful immunodeficiency which translates into an inability to immunize the older subject? The answer to that would appear to be 'no'. However, the work that has been done in man supports the concept of waning immunity.

Tetanus is a relatively rare disease but it is completely preventable. At the present time the most significant mortality is in the over-65s. In a study of the degree of protection against tetanus it was found that less than half of the adults over the age of 60 had protective titres of antibody[21]. The number of young adults who had protective titres was significantly higher, approaching 100%. This difference appears to be related to the immunization record. It would appear that the elderly retain their ability to be immunized by tetanus toxoid and to develop protective titres. The older adults do not reach such high levels of antibody, and the fall in levels is more rapid. This suggests that the elderly do not respond as well to tetanus toxoid, and the difference is accounted for by impaired function of T helper cells[14]. The difference, however, is not significant in terms of protection against tetanus which is the important issue.

Influenza is a major problem in the elderly population carrying a high mortality which rises progressively with advancing age. There have been many studies of the efficacy of influenza vaccination. Some of the studies reported that vaccination was ineffective; however, careful examination of these data reveals that in most instances there was poor matching between immunizing antigens and the epidemic strains. In later studies, when the matching was more accurate, there was adequate protection. My conclusion is that influenza vaccination in older persons is successful in reducing the rate of both hospitalization and mortality.

Closer study of the data reveals that the antibody titres are not as high in the elderly as in younger individuals. Nasal secretory antibody production appears to be adequate. *In vitro* work reveals that activation of B cells by influenza viral antigens is decreased in the elderly. These changes can be partially explained by impaired function of the T helper cells.

The findings with pneumococcal vaccine are very similar. Using the vaccine that contains 14 different antigens, it has been shown that most elderly subjects respond to all and produce significant antibody titres. However, the number of subjects producing a two-fold rise in titre is less in the elderly when compared with the young. Furthermore, there are fewer with protective titres at 1 month after immunization and the decline is earlier and more rapid. Studies of efficacy are limited, but it would appear that the current vaccine is not effective in reducing the incidence of pneumococcal pneumonia or its complications. This is partially due to the limited number of serotypes that are involved, and in some studies the attack rate from the serotypes in the vaccine decreased but were replaced by an increase in frequency of the others, effectively leaving the overall incidence unchanged.

These findings indicate that immunization remains a valid preventive strategy in the older patient. Although ageing results in waning immunity, for most people this is not of such a degree that it reduces the efficacy of vaccination.

Recommended Practice

At the present time it is widely accepted that all adults who are at increased risk from the complications of influenza should be vaccinated. This is interpreted to mean those individuals who have chronic obstructive pulmonary disease or cardiac disease. We have seen that the population over 65 are at increased risk, and it is therefore recommended that all elderly people should be encouraged to receive influenza vaccine each season. The only problem with this recommendation is that there is unlikely to be enough vaccine to go around, but this can be attended to as the demand builds, by increased production.

There is no doubt that tetanus is completely preventable and because of this all individuals, regardless of age, should be aware of their status with regard to tetanus vaccine and ensure that it is current. This means a booster every 10 years, which should not be stopped simply because the person is old.

The situation with regard to pneumococcal vaccination is different. There is no compelling evidence that the morbidity or mortality from pneumococcal pneumonia can be reduced by vaccination. Certainly in the institutional setting this appears to be the case. For these reasons pneumococcal vaccine is not recommended for routine prophylaxis in the elderly. This may change as the new vaccines containing more of the serotypes are tried. Furthermore, work is being done on developing new types of vaccine effective against other components of the pneumococcus capsule and likely to have a much broader specificity.

Tuberculosis remains a significant problem in the elderly, and in fact comprises the most significant group of patients. BCG is not recommended for routine use in the elderly. However, certain preventive measures are in order. It needs to be recognized that the elderly entering old people's institutions are at increased risk of contact and therefore should be carefully screened on entry. The tuberculin status needs to be documented: positive reactors with negative chest radiographs need prophylactic chemotherapy with isoniazid; those reactors with positive chest films need more aggressive therapy; those individuals who fail to react need to have regular, annual, tuberculin testing.

CONCLUSIONS

Infection and immunity are inseparably linked. The immune response wanes in old age, due to the effects of ageing and of various disease states that may be present in the host. There are various age changes, the most notable of which is the involution of the thymus gland beginning shortly after puberty. This results in impaired function of T lymphocytes leading to impaired cell-mediated immunity and impaired modulator functions. The latter is manifest as reduced helper function with reduced antibody response (humoral immunity), and reduced suppressor function with increased auto-antibody production. The immune system also appears to be increasingly stimulated in old age which contributes to the many changes, most notably the increased autoantibodies. The stimulation results from the presence of circulating polyclonal activators like endotoxin. These changes probably result from impaired reticuloendothelial function, from abnormal colonic function and increased bacterial colonization.

The increased colonization that has been reported in old age is linked to various pathophysiological changes of ageing which affect various surfaces or body linings. This produces microenvironments which, together with various institutional environments, put the elderly at increased risk of infection; also the incidence of infections like pneumonia or urinary tract has become increasingly common.

Infection has a higher mortality with advancing age. Some of the reasons for this are obvious, in that one is often dealing with a host who has multiple diseases and minimum reserve in various systems. They are less able to combat the infection and are more likely to suffer decompensation leading to added problems like cardiac failure, brain failure with confusion or incontinence of urine. Another very important factor is that disease may present late due to the impairment of both inflammatory response and homeostasis resulting in the attenuation of classical symptoms.

It is therefore of great importance to take very careful histories and perform meticulous examinations in the older patients, recognizing that disease often presents in an atypical or geriatric manner. The earlier a specific diagnosis is made the better the outcome, and the less the risk of permanent increased dependency.

References

1. Valenti, W. M., Randall, G., Trudell, B. S. and Bentley, D. W. (1978). Factors predisposing to oropharyngeal colonization with Gram-negative bacilli in the aged. *N. Engl. J. Med.*, **298**, 1108–11
2. Horan, M. A., Gulati, R. S., Fox, R. A., Glew, E., Ganguli, L. and Keaney, M. (1984). Outbreak of *Shigella sonnei* dysentery on a geriatric assessment unit. *J. Hosp. Infect.*, **5**, 210–12
3. Puxty, J. A. H., Lenton, J. and Fox, R. A. (1985). Neutrophil function in old age – normal chemiluminescense. (In press)
4. Gulati, R. A., Puxty, J. A. H., Horan, M. A. and Fox, R. A. (1985). The use of the nitroblue tetrazolium test in the diagnosis of infection in old age. (In press)
5. Horan, M. A., Lenton, J. and Fox, R. A. (1985). Combined NBT test and latex bead phagocytosis as a test of neutrophil function. *Mech Ageing Devel.*, **29**, 29–33
6. Finkelstein, M. S., Petkun, W. M., Freedman, M. L. and Antopol, S. C. (1983). Pneumococcal bacteremia in adults. *J. Am. Ger. Soc.*, **31**, 19–27
7. Kay, M. M. B. (1979). In: *Recent Advances in Gerontology*. Ofimo, K., Shimada, K., Iriki, M. and Maeda, D. (eds.). p. 442 Amsterdam: Excerpta Medica
8. Makinodan, T. and Peterson, W. J. (1962). Relative antibody forming capacity of spleen cells as function of age. *Proc. Natl. Acad. Sci. USA*, **48**, 234–8
9. Fox, R. A. (1984). *Immunology and Infection in the Elderly*. (Edinburgh, London, Melbourne and New York: Churchill Livingstone)
10. Bentley, D. W. (1984). In: *Immunology and Infection in the Elderly*. Fox, R. A. (ed.) (Edinburgh, London, Melbourne and New York: Churchill Livingstone)
11. Goidl, E. A., Innes, J. B. and Weksler, M. E. (1976). Immunological studies of ageing II. Loss of IgG and high avidity plaque-forming cells and increased suppressor cell activity in ageing mice. *J. Exp. Med.*, **144**, 1037–48
12. Roberts-Thompson, I. C., Whittinghams, S., Youngchaiyud, U. and MacKay, I. (1974). Ageing, immune responses and mortality. *Lancet*, **2**, 368–70

13. Nagel, J. E., Chrest, F. J. and Adler, W. H. (1981). Enumeration of T lymphocyte subsets by monoclonal antibodies in young and aged humans. *J. Immunol.*, **127,** 2086–8
14. Kishimoto, S., Takahama, T. and Mizumachi, H. (1980). Age related changes in the subsets and functions of human T lymphocytes. *J. Immunol.*, **121,** 1773–80
15. Cohen, P. L. and Ziff, M. (1977). Abnormal polyclonal B cell activators in NZB/NZW F_1 mice. *J. Immunol.*, **119,** 1534–7
16. Horan, M. A. and Fox, R. A. (1984). Ageing and the immune response – a unifying hypothesis. *Mech. Ageing Devel.*, **26,** 165–81
17. Chandra, R. K., Joshi, P., Au,B., Woodford, G. and Chandra, S. (1983). Nutrition and immunocompetence of the elderly. Effect of short-term nutritional supplementation on cell mediated immunity and lymphocyte subsets. *Nutr. Res.*, **2,** 223–32
18. Dontas, A. S., Kasviski, P., Papayouito, P. C. and Marketsos, S. G. (1981). Bacteriuria and survival in old age. *N. Engl. J. Med.*, **304,** 939–43
19. Haley, R. W., Hooton, T. M. and Culver, D. H. (1981). Nosocomial infections in US hospitals, 1975–1976: estimated frequency by selected characteristics of patients. *Am. J. Med.*, **70,** 947–59
20. Puxty, J. A. H., Horan, M. A. and Fox, R. A. (1983). Necropsies in the elderly. *Lancet*, **1,** 1262–4
21. Crossley, K., Irvine, P., Warren, J. P., Lee, B. K. and Mead, K. (1979). Tetanus and diphtheria immunity in urban Minnesota adults. *J. Am. Med. Assoc.*, **242(3),** 485–9

3

Skin Infections in the Elderly

M. F. MUHLEMANN and S. K. GOOLAMALI

INTRODUCTION

The human skin is a reservoir for many different bacteria, the majority of which are non-pathogenic commensals. Changes in the host defence system may allow previously non-pathogenic commensals to become pathogens. An intact skin and mucosal barrier provide an important defence system against infection particularly in the elderly in whom age-related and environmental changes predispose to infection. The aged skin appears dry and wrinkled with a waxy yellowish hue lacking the suppleness of youth. The eccrine and apocrine sweat glands are reduced in number and activity but the sebaceous glands, although less active in post-menopausal women, retain near-optimum function in men in spite of age and are capable of normal function if stimulated by exogenous androgens. Chemical changes in dermal collagen and elastin result in a loss of elasticity. There is also a decrease in blood supply, which in some areas is secondary to peripheral vascular disease.

Normal skin flora include Micrococcaceae, *Proprionibacterium acnes (P. acnes)* and the aerobic diphtheroids. The Micrococcaceae group include micrococci, staphylococci and sarcinia organisms. These bacteria are present in the stratum corneum and the pilosebaceous follicles. The frequency with which these bacteria can be found differs with age but the normal flora of elderly skin consists largely of streptococci, staphylococci and the aerobic diphtheroids[1]. *P. acnes* becomes less abundant with decreased levels of skin lipid which occurs in old age. Both alpha-haemolytic streptococci and non-haemolytic streptococci are found more commonly on elderly skin, whereas

43

the beta-haemolytic streptococci are seldom found on the skin but may be isolated from the throat. Non-pathogenic coagulase-negative staphylococci colonize the skin and the pathogenic coagulase-positive *Staphylococcus aureus* the anterior nares, ears and perineum. Other Gram-negative organisms not infrequently found are regarded by most as temporary residents and may be isolated in many elderly patients. The enteric bacteria found are *Pseudomonas aeruginosa, Escherichia coli,* and *Proteus mirabilis.* The yeast *Candida albicans* is frequently isolated but rarely causes symptoms on healthy skin though is a common pathogen on macerated skin. The dermatophyte fungi are less common than in the young adult.

The skin acts as a dry mechanical barrier and its continual desquamation prevents bacterial colonization. It also exhibits bactericidal properties attributed to the unsaturated fatty acids, in particular oleic acid, produced by bacterial action on skin sebum[2]. Normal commensals may cause bacterial inhibition by the production of antibiotics which limit the growth of potential pathogens[3]. An increase in skin hydration[4] and decrease in skin surface lipid occur in elderly skin, and these may facilitate bacterial colonization. Factors such as obesity, immobility, reduced personal hygiene, malnutrition and a depressed immune response all create favourable circumstances for colonization and a breach of the host's defences.

STREPTOCOCCAL INFECTIONS OF THE SKIN

Haemolytic streptococci are isolated most frequently from the elderly, and not surprisingly are responsible for much skin and subcutaneous infection. The beta-haemolytic group A streptococcus, *S. pyogenes,* is usually found in the pharynx and nose and may be carried for several weeks after an infection. Asymptomatic carriers, especially among medical staff, are a potential source of infection and may be the cause of outbreaks of infection in hospitalized patients. Haemolytic streptococci may also be found colonizing macerated or inflamed skin associated with many dermatoses. *S. pyogenes* is responsible for erysipelas, cellulitis, necrotizing fasciitis and some forms of intertrigo. Repeated local infections may occur as a consequence of impaired lymphatic drainage.

The group A streptococci produce erythrogenic and pyrogenic toxins. The latter are involved in the production of exotoxic shock, myocardial and hepatic damage and can affect reticuloendothelial function and lymphocyte responsiveness. *S. pyogenes* is typed according to its T and M proteins and new strains continue to emerge. Skin disease is principally associated with M types 31, 49, 55–57, 60 and 63.

Erysipelas

Erysipelas is a superficial infection of the skin and lymphatics by *S. pyogenes* and occasionally by groups B, C and G streptococci. The patient with erysipelas is ill with fever, headache and malaise.

Clinical Features

There is a rapidly advancing well-demarcated, often elevated border of erythema and oedema which is extremely tender. The skin appears shiny and tense with peripheral vesiculation and occasional haemorrhage (Figure 3.1). In a study of 329 cases the lower limbs were involved in 67%, the face in 25% and the arms and perineum in 5% and 2.5% respectively[5]. When there is facial involvement the spread is usually in a 'butterfly' distribution across both cheeks and extending onto the forehead (Figure 3.3). With resolution there is desquamation and pigmentation. Common portals of entry are the interdigital toe webs, leg ulcers, minor abrasions and other dermatoses such as eczema and intertrigo. With facial erysipelas the angles of the mouth, nose, ears and inner canthus of the eyes are the main portals.

Diagnosis

In the elderly erysipelas can be a severe and debilitating illness with a poor prognosis if septicaemia is present. Local abscess formation is sometimes a sequel. The immunocompromised patient may present special difficulties in diagnosis as the early morphological clues may be absent or difficult to recognize. The typical erythema may be absent, the eruption may be ill-defined or the oedema may develop long before the pyrexia[6]. Absence of the classical signs in these patients may delay diagnosis and worsen the prognosis. Erysipelas due to groups B, C and G streptococci has been reported in the immunosuppressed patient and may account for some of the atypical signs.

Diagnosis should be confirmed when possible by culture of the bacteria but this may be difficult from the skin lesions, and throat and nasal swabs should also be taken. The diagnosis may also be confirmed serologically by finding raised titres of antideoxyribonuclease B but the antistreptolysin titre is an unreliable guide to recent skin streptococcal infection. Underlying diseases causing immunosuppression should be excluded as must diabetes mellitus. Coexistent dermatoses should be treated to avoid recurrent infection.

Treatment

Treatment should be commenced with penicillin without waiting for bacterial confirmation and the parenteral route may be preferred initially. Recurrent attacks may require prophylactic penicillin. On occasions other organisms may cause erysipelas and these include *Haemophilus influenzae*, *S. pneumoniae* and *Staph. aureus*. Although the diagnosis is seldom difficult, except for those atypical cases associated with immunosuppression, the differential diagnosis should include cellulitis, acute contact dermatitis and drug reactions.

Cellulitis

Cellulitis is an acute or subacute infection of the skin and subcutaneous tissue which may at times be difficult to differentiate from erysipelas. Generally the inflammation of cellulitis is more diffuse and the margins of the erythema less well demarcated. Constitutional symptoms are similar to those of erysipelas although the fever may be less marked. Cellulitis in the elderly is more common on the lower limbs where the aetiology is usually an infected leg ulcer or an abrasion that has been colonized by *S. pyogenes* or *Staph. aureus*. These two organisms account for most cases of cellulitis, though others have caused infection in the immunosuppressed patient.

Clinical Features, Diagnosis and Treatment

The clinical features are those of pain, erythema and swelling. Lymphangitis and lymphadenopathy are less frequently found than with erysipelas. Suppuration, necrosis and gangrene may supervene when the inflammation is intense. Needle aspiration does not significantly aid diagnosis but incision and aspiration of pus may do so. Treatment should be with penicillin combined with a penicillinase-resistant penicillin.

Necrotizing Fasciitis

This is an uncommon condition but frequently affects the elderly and is almost always caused by a group A beta-haemolytic streptococcus. If early and radical surgical treatment is not commenced then the condition carries a grave prognosis.

Clinical Features

First described as haemolytic streptococcal gangrene[7] the disease may present in one of two ways[8]. It may begin with an acute onset of pain and swelling of the skin with a blotchy erythema with indistinct margins. The oedema increases and the skin develops an ominous dusky purple hue of incipient gangrene, with haemorrhagic blistering (Figure 3.2). Constitutional symptoms may be slight at first but rapidly become severe. The alternative presentation may be more insidious with a history of an erysipelas or cellulitis that has failed to respond to conventional antibiotics which then gradually develops necrosis and gangrene. The most common sites to be affected by necrotizing fasciitis are the legs and perineum.

A bacterial necrotoxin is thought to be responsible for the spread of inflammation along the deep fascial planes. Thrombosis develops in the subcutaneous vessels and results in ischaemia and gangrene in the overlying subcutis and cutis. Unfavourable prognostic indicators are a delay in diagnosis, diabetes mellitus, arteriosclerosis, obesity, poor nutrition and age[9]. The mortality is high when diagnosis or treatment has been delayed and in some reports reaches 100%. Death is attributed to hypervolaemic shock with cardiac and renal failure.

Diagnosis

The diagnosis should be considered in any patient with a rapid onset of gangrene or in patients who have failed to respond to adequate antibiotic therapy and in whom gangrene has subsequently developed. The differential diagnoses are the other types of gangrene, particularly gas gangrene and progressive bacterial synergistic gangrene, severe erysipelas and cellulitis. *S. pyogenes* may be cultured from the blister fluid or the necrotic tissue provided there has been no previous antibiotic therapy. Blood culture is usually negative. Frozen section tissue biopsy has been advocated as useful in early diagnosis[10].

Treatment

Surgical debridement is the treatment of choice with postoperative antibiotic cover. Skin grafting is usually required and early grafting and mobilization may improve survival rates[11]. Parenteral nutrition during the acute stages is also thought to improve survival.

STAPHYLOCOCCAL INFECTIONS OF THE SKIN

Staphylococcal skin infection is not as common in old age as in the young in whom it is a frequent pathogen and maybe responsible for bullous impetigo, furunculosis and the syndrome of toxic epidermal necrolysis. The pathogenic strain *Staph. aureus* colonizes the nose and the perineum in symptomatic and asymptomatic carriers but is rarely found on normal skin. It can, however, be regularly isolated from skin lesions of eczema, psoriasis and from leg ulcers. The pathogenicity of the staphylococcus varies toward the skin, and is dependent on the phage types, of which 79 and 80 have been most regularly isolated from lesions of impetigo. *Staph. aureus* can produce leukocidin, coagulase and staphylokinase enzymes and a necrolytic toxin. The most important of these from a clinical standpoint is the epidermolytic toxin which is produced by phage group II bacteria and in particular type 71. This toxin results in the scalded skin syndrome in infants and children, but is rare in adults except perhaps in the immunosuppressed patient. The toxin has also been demonstrated in blister fluid of impetigo[12]. Susceptibility to infection is increased with poor nutrition, alcoholism and immunoparesis. Recurrent infection may be associated with underlying disease or a hitherto unrecognized skin disease.

Impetigo

This is a superficial infection of the skin either by *Staph. aureus* or streptococci. In the elderly the lesions are usually of the bullous type and often occur on the face (Figure 3.4). Recurrent infections may be associated with diabetes mellitus or lymphoproliferative disease. The lesions develop as erythematous macules which rapidly spread and blister. The bullae are superficial and seldom reach any size before they burst leaving honey-coloured 'stuck-on' crusts. Constitutional symptoms are uncommon. Impetigo tends to remain localized but satellite bullae can develop and if untreated may spread rapidly. The epidermolytic toxin causes a plane of cleavage in the stratum corneum and granular layer of the skin with blisters which contain Gram-positive cocci, polymorphs and some acantholytic cells. The differential diagnosis should include pemphigus vulgaris and pemphigus foliaceus, herpes simplex, drug eruptions and eczema.

Treatment

Treatment is with both topical and systemic antibiotics. Topical treatment is with chlortetracycline or neomycin-containing ointments with flucloxacillin or erythromycin given orally.

Carbuncles

This condition is more common in the elderly patient and particularly so in males. A carbuncle is a deep-seated infection of several grouped hair follicles with an intense perifollicular and subcutaneous inflammation. *Staph. aureus* is usually isolated from the lesion. It can occur with other dermatoses or may complicate diabetes mellitus, corticosteroid therapy and cardiac failure. The lesion begins as a firm, painful dome-shaped swelling which can develop up to 10cm in diameter. After a few days suppuration develops, and there is discharge from multiple follicular orifices. Healing occurs with scarring. Constitutional symptoms are marked with high fever and prostration. Therapy with antibiotics, topical antiseptics and analgesics will resolve early small carbuncles but the larger lesions may require surgical incision and drainage.

Erythrasma

Erythrasma may be mistaken for intertrigo, but it is a superficial skin infection by *Corynebacterium minutissimum* which occurs in intertriginous areas. This Gram-positive diphtheroid is part of the normal flora of skin and can be demonstrated in the toe webs of healthy adults. Maceration of the skin promotes bacterial colonization and disease.

Clinical Features and Diagnosis

Erythrasma affects the axillae, groins, submammary and intergluteal skin and is more common in obese patients. An association with diabetes mellitus has been noted. Early lesions consist of well-defined erythematous smooth scaly plaques which become darker and mildly lichenified with time (Figure 3.5). In most patients the lesions are asymptomatic although pruritus is occasionally a feature. Diagnosis is confirmed on culture and with Wood's (longwave) light by the presence of a salmon-pink fluorescence, due to porphyrin-like substances produced by the organism.

Pityriasis versicolor may be mistakenly diagnosed but the lesions are more common on the trunk and fluoresce a pale yellow. Tinea infection of the toe webs and groins may be difficult to differentiate clinically, but they lack fluorescence and there is usually more inflammation present. A pink fluorescence is occasionally found with normal hair follicles on the upper trunk caused by the yeast *Pityrosporum ovale*.

Treatment

Erythrasma responds promptly to systemic erythromycin but topical antibiotics are less effective. Whitfield's ointment (benzoic acid compound, BPC) and the imidazole antifungal creams are effective topical measures.

PARASITIC INFESTATION

Scabies

Problems in diagnosis often arise because of previous inadequate treatment which makes observation of burrows and the isolation of the acarus or its ova difficult. In the elderly, patients in mental institutions, patients with impaired immunosurveillance due to disease or immunosuppressive drugs, infestation may be extensive and the clinical presentation atypical. Burrows are often inapparent and the picture is often that of an exfoliative dermatitis. The typical eruption, however, consists of pruritic papules, vesicles and burrows caused by the ubiquitous mite *Sarcoptes scabiei*. The papules result from invasion of the larval stages of the parasite, the vesicles from host sensitization and the burrow marks the site of the adult female mite where it has dug into the horny layer of the epidermis. In adults the eruption tends to favour the fingerwebs, flexor aspects of the wrists, axillae and the genitalia.

Treatment

The standard procedure for treatment is as follows: Initially the patient takes a hot bath and is told to gently scrub all the skin, except the head, thoroughly. Benzyl benzoate (BPC) (25% emulsion of benzyl benzoate) is painted on all areas of skin from the neck downwards. It is essential that the application includes the axillae, groins, perineum and the toewebs. The skin is left unwashed for 24 hours. The patient then takes a bath and the whole treatment is repeated once more. A total of 120 ml benzyl benzoate is sufficient for both treatments. The main reasons for apparent failure are either inadequate treatment or reinfection by close untreated contacts. It is therefore vital that all persons occupying the same accommodation, as well as other close contacts, should be similarly treated whether or not they show overt evidence of scabies. Even after successful treatment considerable irritation and eczematization may remain for several weeks. This is partly due to the response of the skin to the acarus and its products and partially to treatment. For this, crotamiton ointment, BP (Eurax) with hydrocortisone cream applied two or three times a day is extremely useful. Occasionally scabies may present with marked secondary bacterial infection which should be treated with systemic antibiotics and a topical antibiotic or antiseptic such as Vioform. It is well worthwhile looking closely for pediculosis in patients with scabies since the two are frequently found together.

Pediculosis (Lice)

The incidence of this disease remains high. There are three main types:

pediculosis capitis in which nits are attached to the hair shafts, and lice infest the hair and eyelashes, and which is often complicated by impetigo of the scalp; pediculosis corporis in which the eggs are present on the seams of underclothing; and pediculosis pubis in which the 'crabs' are attached to the base of the pubic hairs. Doubt about the safety of DDT and gamma-benzene hexachloride and the emergence of resistant strains of lice lead to the widespread use of malathion, an organic phosphorus compound, which is now the treatment of choice for pediculosis. A lotion containing 0.5% malathion in 10ml is applied to the head and left *in situ* for 24 hours before being shampooed off. In pediculosis corporis a 1% malathion dusting powder is used on the body and clothes in a similar way. Particular care should be taken to avoid contamination of the eyes.

HERPES ZOSTER

Varicella and herpes zoster have the same aetiology – the varicella zoster virus. During an attack of varicella the virus spreads along peripheral nerves to dorsal root ganglia where it lies dormant until reactivated by trauma, immunosuppressive therapy, development of malignancy or local irradiation (Figure 3.6). In most patients, however, no obvious trigger factor can be identified.

Children in contact with herpes zoster may develop chickenpox. Postherpetic neuralgia complicates zoster in 20–50% of patients over the age of 50 years. The gnawing pain fortunately subsides in the majority but it may take months or even years.

Treatment

Although zoster-immune globulin obtained from healthy adults convalescing from herpes zoster is effective in the prophylaxis of varicella, it has no effect on established zoster infection. Topical idoxuridine 5–40% in DMSO is thought to speed healing and reduce the duration of pain of herpes zoster. It is also said to lessen the incidence of postherpetic neuralgia though opinions vary on this considerably. Systemic corticosteroids appear to reduce the incidence of postherpetic neuralgia in patients over 60 and are indicated in the elderly provided the patient is not already on immunosuppressive therapy. Like idoxuridine, the corticosteroid is best started as soon as the diagnosis is certain, early in the course of the illness. Usually prednisolone is given as a single morning dose of 40–60mg for a week and then tailed off over a period of 3 weeks. In practice, the risk of disseminating zoster is low. More recently acyclovir, a nucleoside analogue, which like idoxuridine inhibits replication of some herpes viruses when given intravenously, has been shown to relieve the acute pain in herpes zoster in the elderly, but does not prevent postherpetic neuralgia[13, 14]. Topical acyclovir is useful in eye infections with zoster virus, improves resolution time, and also reduces the recurrence rate in herpes zoster keratouveitis[15].

Painful trigger zones of postherpetic neuralgia may be relieved by local infiltration of triamcinolone 2mg/ml in procaine or xylocaine. Excision of scarred neuralgic skin can also produce significant pain relief.

CANDIDIASIS

This group of disorders due to the yeast *Candida albicans* or other candida strains is becoming increasingly prevalent, aided by the widespread use of antibiotics and corticosteroids[16]. *Candida albicans* is present normally on the skin or mucous membranes as a commensal, and the development of a positive culture from a swab or scrapings should not be regarded as proof of candida infection. Apart from the clinical appearances, the best confirmatory evidence is demonstration of hyphae by direct microscopy of scrapings or histological section. A number of local or systemic factors favour development of candidiasis (Table 3.1).

Table 3.1 Local and systemic factors in candidiasis

Systemic factors	Local factors
Diabetes mellitus	Intertrigo
Corticosteroid therapy	Topical corticosteroid therapy
Antibiotic therapy	Dentures
Cushing's syndrome	
Old age	
Severe illness	
Addison's disease	
Hypothyroidism	
Iron deficiency	
Pseudohypoparathyroidism	

Treatment

Nystatin and amphotericin B are both highly effective against candidiasis. Frequently candida is superimposed on pre-existing seborrhoeic eczema or flexural psoriasis. It is also common in obese subjects. The eruption should initially be treated with nystatin ointment 3%, applied three times daily, apposed surfaces being separated by non-adherent dressings. When overt candidiasis has cleared, any underlying eczema or psoriasis should be treated. Perianal intertrigo is often associated with intestinal candidiasis. If stool examination confirms the presence of candida, a course of nystatin tablets (500000 units three times daily for 2 weeks) should be given to prevent relapses. Oral candidiasis is most frequently associated with the use of dentures. Presumably the infection is caused by lack of hygiene together with minor trauma to the mucous membranes. Oral ulceration from any cause is frequently secondarily invaded by candida. The treatment of choice is amphotericin B lozenges sucked 4-hourly coupled with maintenance of oral hygiene using regular mouth washes (compound thymol glycerin, BPC). Dentures should be carefully cleaned and sterilized daily and left out at night. Angular stomatitis is commonly due, at least in part, to candida infection and occurs when the cleft of the mouth is deepened by progressive recession of the gingiva in elderly edentulous patients. Nystatin ointment accelerates healing.

Griseofulvin has no effect on *Candida albicans,* though a more recently described imidazole oral antifungal agent ketoconazole has proved useful particularly in long-standing resistant onychomycosis and mucocutaneous candidiasis. This drug is yet to be proved superior than other better-known and well-tried topical preparations for ordinary yeast or dermatophyte skin infections.

RINGWORM

The prevalence of different species of ringworm varies greatly with geographical location. The species can conveniently be classified as anthropophilic (exclusively human parasite) and zoophilic (predominantly animal but facultatively human parasites).

Treatment

For all but the mildest ringworm infection the treatment of choice is griseofulvin. Mild ringworm will respond satisfactorily to Whitfield's ointment (benzoic acid compound ointment, BPC) applied three times daily. Tinea pedis is extremely prevalent. Nevertheless, not all patients with maceration and scaliness between the toes have ringworm. In many it is due to eczema or bacterial infection and no dermatophytes can be isolated from scrapings. Thus whenever possible scrapings should be examined before embarking on fungicidal treatment. If fungus infection is confirmed, and for more severe cases where the sole of the foot is extensively invaded, griseofulvin 500mg daily should be given for 6–8 weeks. Occasionally tinea pedis may present as an acute vesicular eruption. Antibiotic therapy may then be required in addition to griseofulvin if there is secondary bacterial infection.

Tinea corporis should be treated with griseofulvin 500mg daily for 4–6 weeks. Ringworm of the fingernails responds slowly to treatment with griseofulvin which must be continued for at least 6 months. Even then some cases, especially those due to *Trichophyton rubrum,* may fail to respond. For toenails even longer treatment regimes of 1–2 years are required, but it is the experience of most dermatologists that total eradication of ringworm from the toenails is rarely achieved and it is therefore preferable in many cases not to initiate griseofulvin. For the same reason avulsion of the toenails is not to be recommended.

LEG ULCERATION: DIAGNOSIS AND MANAGEMENT

Leg ulceration is predominantly a problem of the middle-aged and elderly. The majority of ulcers are venous but arterial insufficiency is often found. The processes that lead to ulceration are usually irreversible and once ulceration is established recurrence is all too common.

The Postphlebitic Syndrome

This term applies to chronic venous insufficiency of the leg from deep vein thrombosis but similar changes would occur from chronic venous insufficiency from any cause. The changes in the leg result from a sustained rise in venous pressure in the deep or communicating venous systems. This rise in pressure is a result of valvular damage and is transmitted directly to the skin capillary bed. The muscle-pumping action that occurs during exercise produces a fall in the venous pressure recorded in the foot veins from the resting value of 80–100mmHg to 30mmHg. With valvular damage this expected fall does not occur so that the column of blood within the deep veins rises and falls haphazardly and the pressures remain between 80 and 100mmHg. This increased pressure results in capillary elongation, tortuosity and a reduction in dermal capillaries. A decrease in the calf pump efficiency can be correlated with an increased number of capillaries[17], but microscopic studies show an increase in tortuosity rather than in number[18]. Capillary permeability is increased and leakage of plasma occurs into the tissues. Pericapillary fibrin deposition occurs, and there is reported to be a decreased plasma fibrinolytic activity and an elevated serum fibrinogen level in these patients[19]. Experimental model systems show that fibrin is capable of reducing oxygen diffusion, but not that of carbon dioxide. Fibrin cuffing of the capillaries may therefore enhance tissue ischaemia and a defective fibrinolytic system maintains this block. Supporting evidence of the role of fibrin is given by the finding that the fibrinolytic enhancing drug stanozolol can improve some patients with venous lipodermatosclerosis[20]. Ultimately the fibrin is replaced by organized scar tissue and the process is then irreversible.

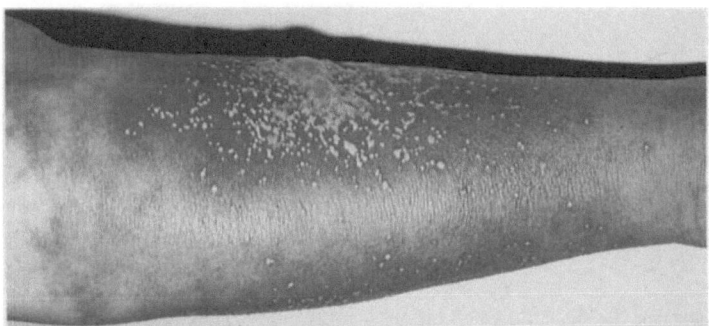

Figure 3.1 Erysipelas on the arm

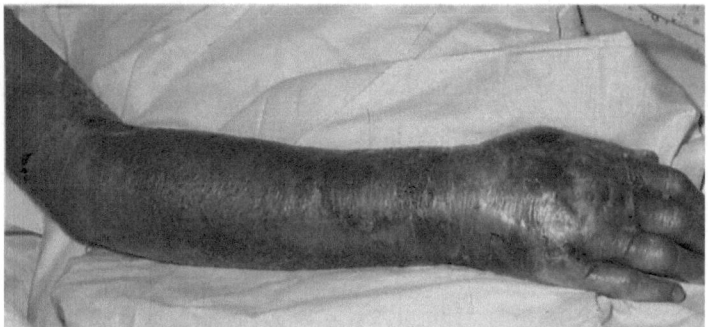

Figure 3.2 Necrotizing fasciitis

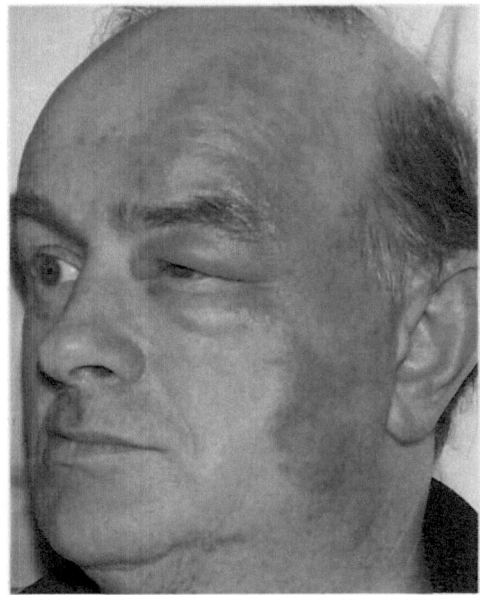

Figure 3.3 Erysipelas on the face

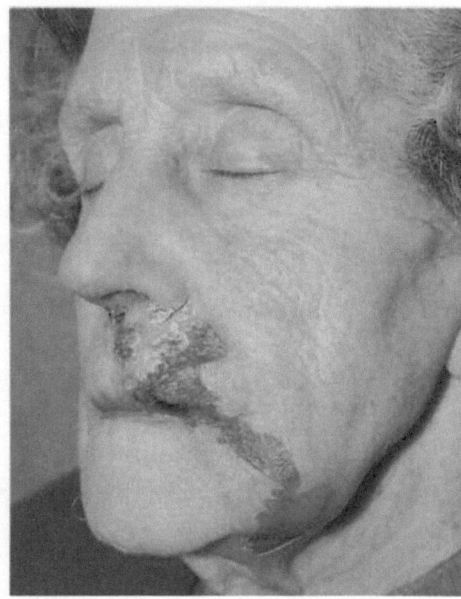

Figure 3.4 Impetigo

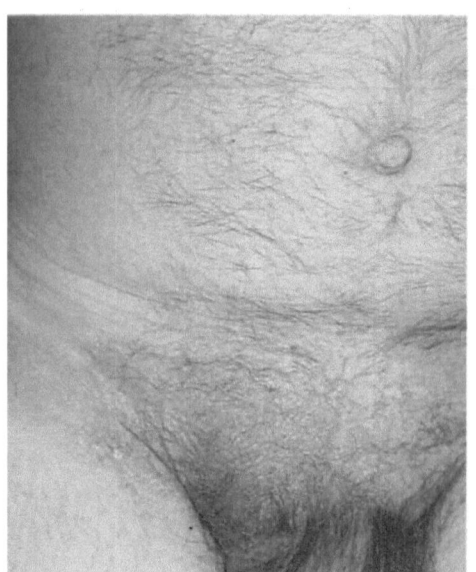

Figure 3.5 Erythrasma

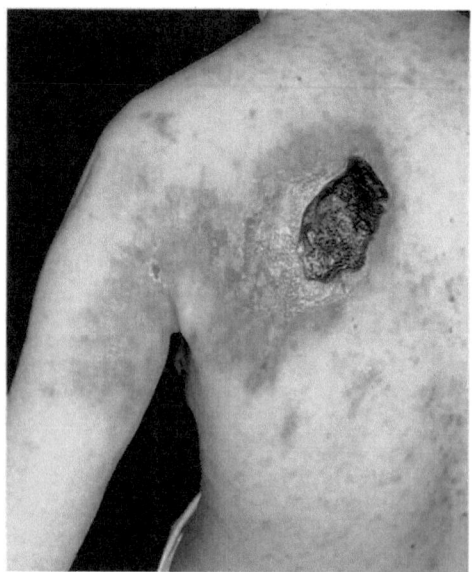

Figure 3.6 Herpes zoster and varicella eruption

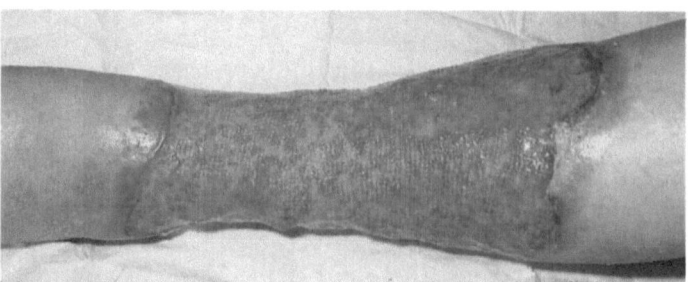

Figure 3.7 Leg ulcer on the calf

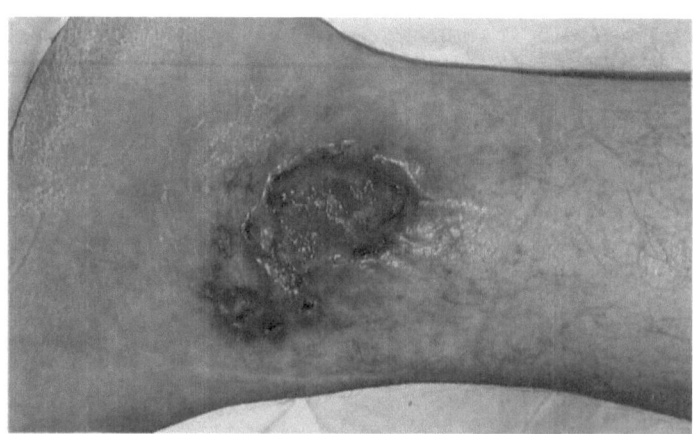

Figure 3.8 Arterial leg ulcer on the ankle

Diagnosis

Pain is not a prominent feature of venous insufficiency, but aching and heaviness in the limbs are frequent complaints. There is usually a mild oedema, haemosiderin deposition with pigmentation, localized eczema and occasionally a capillaritis. Ulceration when it occurs is often a result of minor trauma or recurrent infection. The recurrent inflammation of cellulitis and thrombophlebitis produces progressive sclerosis and secondary lymphoedema.

Venous Ulceration

Ulceration is usually accompanied by changes of chronic venous insufficiency. A history of deep venous thrombosis is obtained in many, but in others it is often assumed that the thrombosis has been silent. Congenital absence of the valves may account for some of these cases. A true varicose ulcer due to incompetence of the superficial saphenous vein alone is uncommon. Venous ulcers are typically at the site of maximum pressure and usually over the inner aspect of the lower calf, the site of the inferior perforating veins. Ulcers can become large, completely encircling the leg and a violaceous and indurated boggy margin are signs of a non-healing ulcer (Figure 3.7). There may be polypoid change surrounding the ulcer which is secondary to capillary hypertrophy and lymphatic block. Serous exudation can be considerable with large ulcers.

Complications

Ulcers are colonized by many strains of bacteria but few of these seem to be of any real significance and evidence that they inhibit tissue healing is lacking. Organisms that are frequently found are *E. coli*, *Proteus mirabilis*, *Pseudomonas aeruginosa* and *Staph. aureus*. Group A beta-haemolytic streptococci warrant prompt treatment with systemic antibiotics, while group G streptococci and *Staph. aureus* may be non-pathogenic in this situation. *Staph. aureus* is sometimes responsible for cellulitis. Eczema is a frequent finding around ulcer sites and is usually a feature of chronic venous insufficiency. A contact allergy may be caused by topical medicaments used on the ulcer. Common sensitizers include topical antibiotics, in particular neomycin, lanolin, colophony and parabens. The eczema may be due to an irritant effect of topical desloughing and antiseptic agents such as benzoyl peroxide and eusol. Dissemination of eczema is not uncommon in such circumstances.

Other complications include haemorrhage, lymphoedema, subcutaneous calcification, periostitis, fibrous ankylosis of the ankle and, rarely, malignant change.

Arterial Leg Ulcers

It is possible to determine clinically if an ulcer is of arterial origin but often there are features of venous insufficiency in addition. Certain historical features and the clinical examination will point to arterial disease as being primarily responsible. Pain is a prominent feature of arterial ulcers especially those associated with areas of white atrophy (Figure 3.8). The ulcers have a punched-out appearance, are often deep and covered by an adherent slough. The margins are indurated and undermined. Chronic cutaneous ischaemia causes a loss of the hair on the dorsal surface of the foot and toes, dryness and atrophy of the skin and a nail dystrophy. The commonest cause of ischaemic ulceration in the elderly is atheromatous disease of the abdominal aorta and limb vessels. Ulceration involving the foot does not occur with pure venous insufficiency, and when present implies arterial or neurological involvement. Ulcers frequently complicate diabetes mellitus as a result of peripheral microvascular disease and neuropathy. The elderly diabetic is particularly vulnerable so that care of the foot is of the utmost importance. Deposition of fibrous tissue around small arterioles occurs with scar tissue formation and areas of radiodermatitis are especially prone to ulceration. Disease of the vessel wall with a polyarteritis may result in ulcers, and if severe a peripheral gangrene. Intermittent claudication and nocturnal rest pain are symptoms associated with advanced major vessel disease and pain is exacerbated by limb elevation and cold. Typically pain relief is achieved by hanging the affected limb out of the bed, but this also results in an increase in the dependent oedema and a worsening of the ischaemia. Cyanosis and a blotchy erythema occur when the circulation is severely compromised and may herald the development of gangrene. Limb elevation also induces extreme pallor and pain with a slow return of colour when released. Fungal infections of the skin and nails are increased with ischaemia.

Some types of ulcers deserve special mention. In the presence of a vasculitis the ulcers are frequently small and numerous. Haemoglobinopathies produce slow-healing ulcers on the shins. Cutaneous tuberculosis and tertiary syphilis uncommon in western Europe may occur in the elderly immigrant population. Systemic sclerosis, Raynaud's disease and systemic lupus erythematosus (SLE) all may give rise to atypical leg ulcers.

Investigation

Healing of an ulcer requires not only careful local treatment but also an assessment of the general physical and social wellbeing of the patient with investigation of the cardiac, renal and hepatic function. A haematological profile and nutritional status is important. The general examination should also include an assessment of the peripheral pulses, the blood pressure, auscultation for arterial bruits and exclusion of xanthomata. Obesity is common in these patients. Reduction in mobility due to arthritis, lung disease or cardiac failure decreases the muscle pump effect and potentiates venous stagnation. Bilateral oedema of cardiac or renal origin increases the skin tension so that minor trauma may precipitate serous discharge and the risk of secondary infection. An anaemia is not uncommon either due to a dietary deficiency of iron or associated with chronic disease. Correction of the anaemia is important as it restores peripheral tissue oxygenation and so promotes healing. Serum zinc levels may be low in some patients with chronic ulcers, but views of the precise role of zinc replacement therapy in ulcer healing are conflicting. Every encouragement should be given to mobilize the patient with avoidance of prolonged periods of limb dependency which aggravate the oedema.

Simple investigations should be carried out on all patients with leg ulcers and should include a blood count, electrolytes, blood sugar, and, where appropriate, a chest X-ray and e.c.g. With atypical ulceration the investigation should be extended to include protein and haemoglobin electrophoresis, syphilis serology, autoantibody screening, cryoglobulins, and skin biopsy. Non-invasive assessment of blood flow by the doppler technique and arteriograms are usually necessary if surgery is contemplated.

Treatment

An understanding of the aetiology is important as certain aspects of therapy depend on the cause. Topical measures are applicable to both venous and arterial ulcers. At the earliest possible stage venous insufficiency should be treated by compression bandaging or elasticated stockings. Surgical intervention and correction of communicating vein incompetence may prevent later venous ulceration. However, once this has occurred compression bandaging is mandatory to provide a counter pressure to support the leg, and to prevent capillary leakage with its subsequent problems. Pressure bandaging enables the patient to remain ambulatory. Periods of bedrest are sometimes necessary for relief of pain and treatment of oedema, but it must be weighed against the risks of ankle fixation and possible further deep venous thrombosis. Clearly, strong compression must be avoided with arterial ulcers as an ischaemic crisis may be precipitated.

Several different types of bandage are now available and the choice is largely an individual one although history of previous allergic sensitivity will preclude some forms of treatment. A popular choice is the zinc oxide occlusive dressing applied from mid-foot to below knee. These are covered by an elastic bandage or by a diachylon bandage for those with a colophony sensitivity. Zinc oxide bandages may be plain or used in combination with clioquinol, calamine or ichthammol. Dressings can be left undisturbed for up to a week, although it is worth checking initially after a few days for possible allergic sensitivity. This type of dressing is unsuitable if there is excessive exudation or heavy bacterial colonization and these would need treatment first. Compression bandages may be used without the paste underbandage, and here again the range of products is large and the choice will depend on the tensile strength required. It is worth noting that some of the strongest will be too strong to be managed by the weaker patient so that dressings will need supervision. Where there is poor arterial flow the weaker elasticated crepe bandages will have to suffice.

Treatment of infection is important although systemic antibiotics are usually only necessary for group A beta-haemolytic streptococcal infection and sometimes *Staph. aureus*. Topical antibiotics may be used for short periods only as the risk of allergic sensitization is increased when they are used for leg ulcers. Neomycin is a recognized sensitizer and cross-sensitivity may occur. Silver sulphadiazine (Flamazine) is a useful topical antibacterial for the treatment of *Pseudomonas aeruginosa* and for prophylaxis against *Staph. aureus*. A dilute solution of acetic acid (3%) is effective against *P. aeruginosa* but can sting on application. Topical antiseptics are frequently used for their antibacterial properties and those of value include povidone-iodine and chlorhexidine. They can be used to cleanse the ulcers and are applied as dressings or used as soaks. Four other antiseptics deserve mention. Hydrogen peroxide (5–7%) in an aqueous solution, potassium permanganate (1 in 8000) solution and benzoyl peroxide are all oxidizing agents which are widely used as dressings and soaks. Edinburgh solution of lime (eusol) is a chlorinated lime and boric acid solution which may be used alone or with liquid paraffin and is particularly useful as a cleansing and desloughing agent. Prolonged use may inhibit granulation tissue formation, and it can cause systemic toxicity if used on large areas of injured skin due to absorption of boric acid. There are advocates for the use of hydroscopic agents to remove cellular debris but these are probably of no greater advantage than agents such as eusol or benzoyl peroxide and generally more expensive.

Improvement of the peripheral circulation is a desirable ideal but there is little evidence that vasodilators have any lasting benefit. Sympathectomy, local heat and alcohol in 'medicinal' quantities produce the best vasodilatation. Drugs which have an effect on red cells and capillaries may be useful in the preulcer and ulcer states. Oxypentifylene has an effect on the deformability of red cells, and has been shown to improve the claudicating distance in patients with peripheral vascular disease, and could be useful in patients with arterial ulcers[21]. The rutosides are said to improve capillary permeability and stanozolol acts as a fibrinolytic agent, both of which are advocated in the therapy of venous insufficiency and ulceration. However, larger clinical trials are necessary to assess the benefits of these drugs in the treatment of ulceration.

Split skin and pinch grafts will speed healing once the ulcers are clean with healthy granulation tissue and free from infection. The survival of these grafts is improved if there has been prior vascular surgery to improve blood supply. This may be achieved by sympathectomy, endarterectomy or reconstructive surgery. The result of pinch grafting for venous ulcers is depressingly poor if no account is taken of the predisposing factors, and some form of compression bandage must be applied as a long-term prophylaxis.

References

1. Sommerville, D. (1969). The effects of age on the normal bacterial flora of the skin. *Br. J. Dermatol.*, **81**, Suppl. **1**, 14–22
2. Ricketts, C. R., Squire, J. R. and Topley, E. (1951). Human skin lipids with particular reference to self sterilising power of skin. *Clin. Sci.*, **10**, 89–111
3. Selwyn, S. (1975). Natural antibiosis among skin bacteria as a primary defence against infection. *Br. J. Dermatol.*, **93**, 487–493
4. Rothman, S. (1954). *Physiology and Biochemistry of the Skin*. (Chicago: University of Chicago Press)
5. Voigtlander, V. (1975). Das erysipel an der Universitats-Hautkliniek Heidelburg 1960–1973. *Z. Hautkrankheit.*, **50**, 135
6. Cupps, T. R., Cotton, D. J., Schooley, R. T. and Fauei, A. S. (1981). Facial erysipelas in the immunocompromised host. *Arch. Dermatol.* **117**, 47–9
7. Meleney, F. L. (1924). Haemolytic streptococcal gangrene. *Arch. Surg.*, **9**, 317
8. Leppard, B. J. and Seal, D. V. (1983). The value of bacteriology and serology in the diagnosis and treatment of necrotizing fasciitis. *Br. J. Dermatol.*, **109 (1)**, 37–44
9. Majewski, J. A. and Alexander, J. W. (1983). Early diagnosis nutritional support and immediate extensive debridement improve survival of necrotizing fasciitis. *Am. J. Surg.*, **145 (6)**, 784–787
10. Stamenkovic, I. and Lew, P. D. (1984). Early recognition of potentially fatal necrotizing fasciitis (the art of frozen section biopsy). *N. Engl. J. Med.*, **310**, 1689–93
11. Percival, R. and Hargreaves, A. W. (1982). Necrotizing fasciitis an alternative approach. *Postgrad. Med. J.*, **58**, 756–9
12. Baker, D. H., Dimond, R. L. and Kirk, D. W. (1978). The epidermolytic toxin of *Staphylococcus aureus*. Its failure to bind to cells and its detection in blister fluid of patients with bullous impetigo. *J. Invest. Dermatol.*, **71 (4)**, 274–5
13. Bean, B., Braun, C. and Balfour, H. H. Jr. (1982). Acyclovir therapy for acute herpes zoster. *Lancet*, **2,** 118–21
14. Peterslund, N. A., Seyer-Hansen, K., Ipsen, J., Esmann, V., Schonheyder, H. and Juhl, H. (1981). Acyclovir in herpes zoster. *Lancet*, **2**, 827–30
15. McGill, J. and Chapman, C. (1983). A comparison of topical acyclovir with steroids in the treatment of herpes zoster keratouveitis. *Br. J. Ophthalmol.*, **2,** 746–50
16. Oriel, J. D., Partridge, B. M., Denny, M. J. *et al*. (1972). Genital yeast infections. *Br. Med. J.*, **4,** 761–4
17. Burnand, K. G., Whimster, I. W., Clemenson, G., Lea Thomas M. and Browse, N. L. (1981). The relationship between the number of capillaries in the skin of the venous ulcer bearing area of the lower leg and the fall in foot vein pressure during exercise. *Br. J. Surg.*, **68,** 297–300
18. Ryan, T. J. (1969). The epidermis and its blood supply in venous disorders of the legs. *Trans. St John's Hosp. Dermatol. Soc.*, **55,** 51–63

19. Burnand, K. G. and Browse, N. L. (1982). The post-phlebitic leg and venous ulceration. In: Russell, R. C. G. (ed) *Recent Advances in Surgery 11*. (Edinburgh: Churchill Livingstone)
20. Burnand, K. G., Clemenson, G., Morland, M., Jarrett, P. E. M. and Browse, N. L. (1980). Venous lipodermatosclerosis: treatment by fibrinolytic enhancement and elastic compression. *Br. Med. J.,* **280,** 7–11
21. Porter, J. M., Cutler, B. S., Lee, B. Y. *et al.* (1982). Pentoxifylline efficacy in the treatment of intermittent claudication. *Am. Heart J.,* **104,** 66–72

4

Septicaemia and Infective Endocarditis

R. K. T. WILLIAMS and M. J. DENHAM

PART 1   SEPTICAEMIA

Septicaemia continues to be a significant cause of morbidity and mortality in all age groups. However, excluding immunosuppressed patients, it is the elderly who are most at risk. This is because of the non-specific way in which many old people present and the multiple, often serious pathologies which coexist in the elderly person.

Bacteraemia, septicaemia and toxaemia are often used interchangeably to describe the same clinical setting and this can lead to some confusion. It has been suggested[1] that bacteraemia should be used where bacteria are present in the bloodstream without clinical illness, septicaemia should be used where bacteria are present and producing signs and symptoms of illness, and toxaemia where bacterial toxins are present in the bloodstream, and producing signs of illness. In practice, these definitions are of limited value in the elderly because the symptoms of multiple disorders will blur any distinction between bacteraemia and septicaemia, and in addition few centres are able to measure toxin levels routinely.

Incidence

Establishing the true incidence of septicaemia is difficult due to differences in definitions of disease used and variations in populations studied, but recent studies have consistently demonstrated a rise in the incidence of septicaemia over the last 30 years[2-4]. Some of the increase is due to greater

61

use of invasive diagnostic instrumentation such as cystoscopy, and this may also account for the greater incidence of septicaemia seen in males in some series[5, 6]. The incidence varies between 0.3% and 0.7% of all hospital admissions[2, 3, 7]. Not surprisingly a higher incidence rate of 1.4% is found in elderly people[8].

Gram-negative organisms form a greater proportion of septicaemias than previously[4, 9–12] particularly in the elderly[13]. However staphylococci and streptococci still cause significant numbers[4, 8, 9, 14].

Mortality

Mortality in septicaemia remains high, despite the intensive treatment now available, and is higher in shocked patients. Other risk factors include the causative agent, infections acquired in hospital, certain drugs such as steroids, and old age [4, 15]. Actual mortality rates vary according to the population studied, but rates of 15–25% are quoted most frequently, rising to 50% in the presence of shock[7, 13, 16, 17]. Death may occur rapidly as a result of cardiac arrest due to severe metabolic disturbance and hypotension. At a later stage, death may be due to secondary end organ damage such as severe lung damage or renal failure[18].

Predisposing Factors

Old age is sometimes given as a predisposing factor to septicaemia[15]. However, it is really the multiplicity of diseases that often occur together, with advancing years, that partly account for the occurrence of septicaemia in the older age groups. In addition, changes in humoral and cell-mediated immunity in older people play a part in decreased resistance to bacterial infection (see Chapter 2).

A focus of infection from which bacteria can gain entry to the bloodstream is obviously the primary predisposing factor, and the lungs, genitourinary tract and biliary tract are the most common portals of entry in the elderly[8, 13, 17].

Secondary factors, such as malignancy or immunosupressive therapy, increase liability to develop a primary focus, but this will apply to all age groups. Investigative or therapeutic instrumentation can precipitate bacteraemia and in these cases natural defences such as the skin and mucous membranes are breached and allow invasion of the bloodstream by commensal bacteria. Procedures such as endoscopy, colonoscopy, sigmoidoscopy, rectal examination and liver biopsy have all been shown to cause bacteraemia[19–23]. However these episodes of bacteraemia are not accompanied by any disturbance to the patient, and prophylactic antibiotics are not indicated except possibly in those with heart valve disease[24]. On the other hand urinary catheterization, cystoscopy and peripheral and arteriovenous cannulae are known to cause septicaemia, and in the case of cystoscopy, appropriate antibiotic cover should be given to those at risk. Increasing numbers of elderly people have implants, such as cardiac pacemakers and joint prostheses, and these sometimes become infected and act as a focus for septicaemia (Chapter 8). Primary, secondary and iatrogenic predisposing factors are shown in Table 4.1.

Table 4.1 Factors predisposing to the development of septicaemia

Primary

Urinary tract infections
Cholangitis
Chest infections
Bowel ischaemia and perforation
Ischaemic ulcers, pressure ulcers and cellulitis
Trauma and burns

Secondary

Malignant disease
Steroid therapy
Cytotoxic therapy and radiotherapy
Lymphomas and myeloproliferative disorders
Hepatic cirrhosis
Diabetes mellitus
Rheumatoid arthritis
Uraemia

Iatrogenic

Cystoscopy and catheterization
Intravenous cannulae
Endoscopic retrograde cholangiopancreatography (ERCP)
Joint prostheses
Pacemaker implants

Microbiology

Table 4.2 shows the organisms most frequently found in septicaemic patients. The bacteria found often reflect the source of infection and may be a clue to the source especially in the absence of appropriate clinical features[13, 17]. Thus *Escherichia coli* would point to the genitourinary and biliary systems, and streptococci to the lungs. Indeed blood culture is often positive when sputum culture is negative[25]. In 20% of cases the source of infection never becomes clear[8, 26]. Occasionally the organism may indicate a more serious underlying condition. Isolation of *Streptococcus bovis* should prompt a search for underlying gastroenterological malignancy[27]. Table 4.3 shows the distribution of bacteria found on blood culture from four studies of patients over 65 years of age, totalling 207 patients[8, 11, 13, 17].

Table 4.2 Organisms which commonly cause septicaemia

Gram-positive organisms

Streptococcus pneumoniae
Staphylococcus aureus
Haemolytic streptococci

Gram-negative organisms

Escherichia coli
Klebsiella aerogenes
Proteus spp.
Pseudomonas pyocyanea
Bacteroides fragilis

Table 4.3 Combined incidence of different bacteria from four studies on septicaemia (207 patients)

Bacterium	Percent
Escherichia coli	43.0
Streptococcus pneumoniae	17.0
Staphylococcus aureus	10.0
Klebsiella pneumoniae	7.7
Beta-haemolytic streptococci	7.2
Proteus spp.	5.3
Streptococcus viridans	2.8
Pseudomonas aeruginosa	1.4

Pathology

Septicaemic shock is due to the damaging actions of exotoxins and endotoxins at a cellular level and the body's response to this damage. In general any organ may be affected, usually with microthrombus formation leading to tissue necrosis and haemorrhage. The kidney and lungs are most at risk due to their large blood flow and susceptability to hypotension[28]. In the kidneys, fibrin thrombi are found in the glomeruli in the early stages with either cortical or tubular necrosis occurring bilaterally as the disease progresses. In the liver, zonal necrosis and fibrin thrombi occur, which may lead to decreased ability of the Kupffer cells to inactivate endotoxins from the colon, thus exacerbating the shock. There is seldom, however, clinical evidence of liver failure[28].

In the lungs the injury occurs in three stages. During the first to third days there is an exudate phase with oedema, haemorrhage, interstitial inflammation and early hyaline membrane formation due to necrosis of type I pneumocytes. A proliferative phase occurs at 3–10 days during which there is proliferation of type II pneumocytes to cover the denuded alveolar surface. The microvasculature is obstructed and compressed. A final fibrotic phase occurs with fibrous tissue forming in the hyaline membranes and alveolar septae[29]. Whether the microthrombi formed are primary or secondary is not clear[30]. Other organs that may be affected are the heart, with subendocardial and muscle necrosis, and the intestine with thrombi and necrosis similar to ischaemic colitis[28]. Haemorrhage may also occur in the pancreas and adrenal glands.

Pathophysiology

The major cause of death in septicaemia is shock, which in Gram-negative septicaemia raises the mortality from 10% in non-shocked patients to 60% in shocked patients[31]. Shock can be defined as the inability of the circulatory system to meet the needs of tissues for oxygen and nutrients and the removal of toxic metabolites[32].

Shock is produced in Gram-positive infections, such as those caused by pneumoccocci, clostridia and staphylococci, by exotoxins. Gram-negative shock is produced by endotoxins. Gram-positive organisms probably account for one-third of the cases of shock with Gram-negative organisms accounting for the remainder, although shock has been described in septicaemia due to almost all bacterial species[33]. Staphylococcal infection can cause the toxic shock syndrome (TSS), usually without obvious bacteraemia. Although commonly associated with menstruating women, the toxic shock syndrome can occur in either sex at any age[34]. Toxic shock syndrome is probably due to circulating staphylococcal exotoxins[35] and should be suspected if there is high temperature, rash with desquamation, hypotension and evidence of either clinical or laboratory involvement of at least three organ systems [36, 37]. Pathological findings in fatal cases include hyaline membrane formation in the lungs, periportal liver inflammation and acute tubular necrosis[38].

The endotoxins which cause Gram-negative septicaemic shock are lipid-A molecules and are attached to cell membranes. Their toxicity is due to the ability of the unusual fatty acids attached to lipid A molecules to penetrate cell and mitochondrial membranes[31]. Endotoxaemia may occur on breakdown of the bacteria or from entry of large quantities of endotoxin into the portal systems from the colon. This results in fever and production of prostaglandins, catecholamines, bradykinin and histamine. Fever is sometimes absent in the elderly for reasons which are not clear. Certainly leukocyte pyrogen, which is produced by mononuclear phagocytes and is responsible for mediation of fever, is normal in the healthy elderly[39].

At a cellular level, peripheral vascular shunting occurs and therefore cellular metabolism proceeds anaerobically with production of large quantities of lactate. Endotoxins also activate the complement system leading to coagulation and fibrinolysis[40]. Initially, the release of bradykinin and histamine leads to vasodilatation and raised cardiac output. The body's response is to increase neural drive to the heart and lungs, resulting in increased heart rate and myocardial contractility. Systemic and pulmonary vasoconstriction then follow, partly due to the high levels of circulating noradrenaline. There is also activation of the renin/angiotensin system and increased levels of glucocorticoids and antidiuretic hormone. These changes lead to further tissue anoxia and pooling in the capillary bed. Damage to endothelial linings leads to extravasation of plasma into tissues. Eventually cardiac output falls and acidosis increases still further, with anoxia and collapse of coronary, renal and cerebral circulation. The situation is then irreversible and death follows quickly.

Four different types of septicaemic shock have been recognized[41]; while they provide a useful classification, the category into which any particular patient falls probably represents the severity of the infection and the point in the disease course at which the diagnosis is made rather than separate clinical syndromes. The categories proposed by McLean[41] are as follows.

Type 1

These patients have a high central venous pressure (CVP), raised blood volume, raised cardiac ouput and alkalosis. Despite this, hypotension is present with warm peripheries and there is lactic acid production and oliguria. Hyperventilation (probably resulting in the alkalosis) is an early sign. Prognosis is good.

Type II

Patients have a high CVP and markedly increased cardiac output, with hyperventilation and restlessness. Peripheral resistance is reduced but hypotension is a late feature. Oliguria is present with a marked lactic acidosis and lactic acidaemia. Prognosis is poor.

Type III

Patients have a low CVP with reduced cardiac output, but this increases with fluid replacement. Alkalosis or a normal pH are present with moderately elevated lactate levels. Oliguria and hypotension are present before treatment. Prognosis is reasonably good provided that treatment results in restoration of a normal blood pressure and urine flow.

Type IV

Patients have a low CVP, low blood volume and low cardiac output which is unresponsive to therapeutic manoeuvres. There is marked acidosis with high lactate levels. Prognosis is poor.

A simplified version of the prognostic features appears in Table 4.4.

Table 4.4 Prognositic features in septicaemic shock

Good prognosis

Alkalosis
High cardiac output
Low cardiac output which responds to treatment

Poor prognosis

Acidosis
Low cardiac output resistant to treatment

Septicaemia without shock can also have profound effects on the lungs, kidneys and coagulation systems. In the lungs, septicaemia is a major cause of the adult respiratory distress syndrome (ARDS). The degree of direct injury to the endothelium by endotoxins is minimal[31], but undoubtedly leads to severe damage. There must therefore be an amplification process which probably involves release of intracellular inflammatory agents, microvascular changes and altered surfactant levels, either decreased production or increased destruction. The changes produced in the alveoli initially cause hypoxaemia with respiratory alkalosis: the chest X-ray is normal. The combination of microthrombi and decreased surfactant levels result in transudation, increased lung compliance and further hypoxia. The chest X-ray shows pulmonary oedema. Damage to the lungs may be extensive and irreversible with atelectasis[30]. Thrombocytopenia may herald the development of ARDS by 24 hours[18].

Renal involvement is usual in septicaemia and is manifested by oliguria. The renal failure can be either prerenal or due to cortical or tubular necrosis[42]. Recovery is usual from prerenal or acute tubular necrosis, but cortical necrosis may require long-term dialysis or transplantation if the patient survives[1]. Estimation of serum and urinary sodium and osmolality is helpful in distinguishing the prerenal from renal causes. In prerenal failure the urinary sodium is low (less than 20mmol/l) and the serum/urine osmolality ratio of higher than 1.5:1. In acute tubular necrosis the urinary sodium will be above 60mmol/l and the serum/urine osmolality ratio 1:1. Cortical necrosis will either be anuric or similar to acute tubular necrosis.

Septicaemia can cause a range of coagulation abnormalities. The exact incidence of these is difficult to determine but Kreger *et al.*[15] estimated that coagulation abnormalities occurred in 64% of Gram-negative septicaemias and that 10% of these had evidence of disseminated intravascular coagulation (DIC). DIC is initiated by endotoxins causing vasoconstriction and damaging vascular endothelium. They also damage platelets, activate Factor XII[43] and, by damaging white blood cells, release neutrophil procoagulant. The resultant formation of microthrombi is exacerbated by the presence of metabolic acidosis and shock[31]. When the thrombotic process starts, the body's fibrinolytic processes attempt to counteract it. If the fibrinolytic factors are consumed faster than they can be generated then a bleeding diathesis can occur which is exacerbated by the action of fibrin degration products (FDP) on fibrin[44]. Disseminated intravascular coagulation is diagnosed by both clinical and laboratory methods. If the platelet count is low, prothrombin time and activated partial thromboplastin time prolonged and fibrinogen levels decreased, then DIC is likely. Other useful parameters are tests for fibrin monomers and fibrin degradation products[15], but it is not clear whether DIC itself contributes to the mortality or whether it merely reflects the severity of the illness.

Clinical Features

Septicaemia usually presents as a severe illness with high fever. However, as is often the case in the elderly, septicaemia can present more subtly. Presentation is often non-specific, causing delay in diagnosis[45]. General malaise, confusion, altered consciousness levels, falls and immobility are common presenting symptoms in the elderly[8, 13, 25]. Other features are hyperventilation (which may mimic pulmonary emboli), hypotension, jaundice, nausea and vomiting. Fever may be mild or even absent and rigors are also less common in the elderly[13, 17].

Features of the history and symptoms can suggest the source of a septicaemic infection. Thus septicaemia with jaundice is likely to be due to biliary infection[13]. While recent incontinence might suggest a urinary tract infection, recent onset of pain in joints, particularly those which have been subject to operation, suggest possible osteomyelitis[8].

As the disease progresses the classical features of hypotension, oliguria and shock may develop. The skin may be warm or cold and moist, but this is a poor guide to the circulatory state[41]. Attempts to distinguish clinically between Gram-positive and Gram-negative septicaemia have been made, but it is now thought that this is not usually possible[16]. Occasionally elderly patients can tolerate bacteraemia with endotoxaemia with no apparent ill-effect[46]. Clinical situations which may be due to septicaemia in the elderly are shown in Table 4.5.

Table 4.5 Clinical situations where there should be a high index of suspicion of septicaemia

Confusion
Altered conscious level
Pyrexia
Unexplained vomiting and diarrhoea
Jaundice
Falls and immobility
Unexplained illness in a patient with prosthetic joint or pacemaker
General malaise
Respiratory symptoms

Investigations

Blood cultures are mandatory in suspected cases of septicaemia. In practice, this means that blood cultures should be part of the routine investigations in any elderly person who is generally unwell. Care needs to be taken in the interpretation of the results as contamination from disinfectants, blood tubes and even the bottles themselves may occur[47-49]. However, with newer laboratory techniques, contamination is uncommon and organisms sometimes regarded as contaminants, such as *Staphylococcus epidermidis,* should not be dismissed without careful thought[50].

Haematological and biochemical investigations may yield useful clues, especially when the clinical diagnosis is not clear. An unexpectedly raised white blood count in any elderly person should lead to blood cultures being taken. Rarely, the white blood count may be low[25] and is usually due to previous chemotherapy[13, 15]. The haemoglobin and urea are of less value. A chest X-ray and a mid-stream or catheter specimen of urine should be taken routinely as clinical signs of urinary tract or chest infection may be absent. Liver function tests may be useful. The transaminases and alkaline phosphatases are often raised in septicaemia[13, 51] and a raised bilirubin is indicative of biliary tract sepsis[8, 13]. Blood sugar estimation is worthwhile as this can fall in severe endotoxaemia due to depletion of glycogen stores and increased utilization of glucose by the tissues[31]. Blood gas analysis should also be performed to detect acidosis, and this may help in predicting outcome[31].

Other tests are of limited value. The *Limulus* test has been used for detection of endotoxin, but lack of sensitivity and specificity limit its usefulness[52]. Similarly the buffy coat smear test detects bacteraemia rapidly, but the concentration of bacteria required to give a positive result predicts 100% mortality[53].

Management and Treatment

Early, vigorous treatment with antibiotics, circulatory and respiratory support, and surgical drainage or removal of septic foci will reduce mortality. However, in the very old, this vigorous approach has to be balanced against underlying disease and premorbid general health.

Antibiotics usually need to be started blind once a diagnosis of septicaemia has been made. Close collaboration between clinician and microbiologist is essential. The choice of antibiotics will vary with local drug resistance problems, antibiotic policies, and the original site of infection (where known), and whether the infection is community-acquired or hospital-acquired. Gentamicin has been the mainstay of treatment, but resistance is quite common [54]. In the elderly, it is also more hazardous as renal damage and ototoxicity occur more readily. Firstline treatment in severe septicaemic shock should be with a combination of cefuroxime, gentamicin and metronidazole given intravenously, at least for the first 24 hours. This combination will cover most likely organisms. Where the clinical presentation suggests a likely site of infection and the patient is less severely ill, a more selective choice of antibiotics can be employed (Table 4.6). Once the infecting organism is known, the choice of antibiotic can be altered with the advice of the microbiologist.

Table 4.6   Antibiotic choice where there is a likely site of infection

Site of infection	Likely organism	Antibiotic
Genitourinary tract	*Escherichia coli*	ampicillin + gentamicin
Biliary tract	*Escherichia coli* anaerobes	ampicillin + gentamicin + metronidazole
Gastrointestinal tract	Gram-negatives + anaerobes	ampicillin + gentamicin + metronidazole
Respiratory infection Community-acquired	*Streptococcus pneumoniae*	Benzylpenicillin
Hospital-acquired	Gram-positive and Gram-negative organisms	cefuroxime
Skin	streptococci and staphylococci	Penicillin and flucloxacillin
Bone and joint infection	*Staphylococcus aureus*	flucloxacillin and fucidic acid

Sources of infection should be eliminated where possible, for example, removal of catheters and drainage of pus with excision of devitalized tissues. However, if the patient is severely ill or the suspected focus is in the bowel, management becomes more difficult. No strict guidelines can be given, but close and early collaboration between physician, microbiologist, anaesthetist and surgeon is essential.

If patients require intensive therapy then they should be transferred to an appropriate care unit. Here treatment of circulatory, renal and respiratory collapse can be carried out with the necessary monitoring techniques. Hypoxaemia may need treatment with increased inhaled oxygen concentrations and if ARDS develops IPPV or PEEP may be necessary[55]. Correction of acidosis and electrolyte disturbances may be carried out, as well as correction of hypovolaemia using central venous and pulmonary wedge pressures. Mannitol or frusemide may help in maintaining urine flow, and adrenergic agents such as dopamine and dobutamine may be required to improve cardiac output. Renal failure is treated in the usual way, but may need dialysis.

Disseminated intravascular coagulation will be present in most patients but few will require treatment[15]. If treatment is necessary, heparin or fresh frozen plasma and platelet infusions may be used, depending on whether haemorrhage or thrombosis predominates. The help of a haematologist is invaluable. Steroids are now thought to be of no benefit in DIC[15, 55]. Similarly, high-dose methyl prednisolone has been used in the treatment of ARDS due to septicaemia, but this has not led to any increase in survival[29]. H_2-antagonists are thought to be of value for reducing stress ulceration. Two new developments may prove useful in future. Prostaglandins play a part in the evolution of endotoxic shock[56], and animal experiments have shown a decrease in mortality in septicaemia, using indomethacin[57]. Human studies are awaited. Another potential exciting development is the use of human antiserum to endotoxin. This has been shown to substantially reduce deaths due to Gram-negative septicaemia in humans[58].

PART II INFECTIVE ENDOCARDITIS

Infective endocarditis is perhaps one of the most difficult illnesses to recognize in the elderly because of its protein manifestations and the wide spectrum of severity at presentation. These factors contribute to the significant mortality which is still found in this disease. The wide range of clinical presentations is largely unrelated to causative organisms and therefore distinction into acute and subacute endocarditis has fallen into disuse.

Incidence and Mortality

It is likely that the incidence of infective endocarditis is relatively unchanged from the preantibiotic era of the 1930s[1]. However, the age distribution has changed dramatically in the last 50 years with the majority of cases now over 50 years of age and a large proportion over 60 years. Thus only 3% of patients with endocarditis were over 60 in 1945 compared to 55% over 60 in 1977[2,3](Figure 4.1). This rise has occurred due to greater longevity of the population as a whole, a decrease in the incidence of rheumatic heart disease and greater life expectancy of those who have rheumatic heart disease, and an increase in the use of invasive instrumentation and procedures. This trend

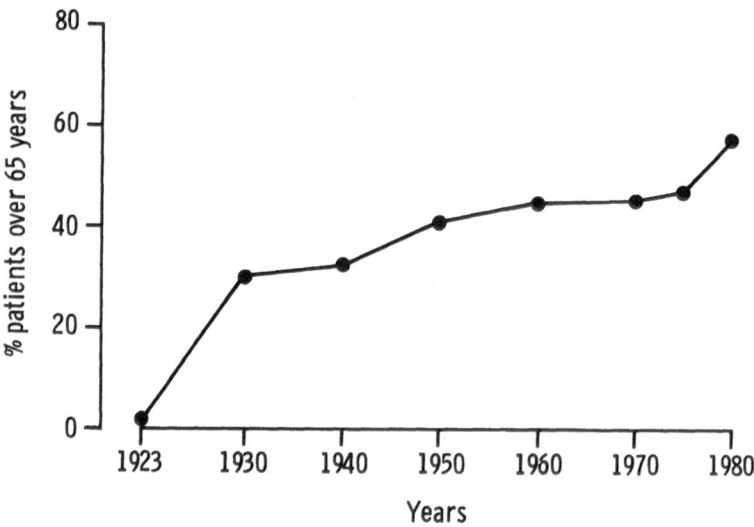

Figure 4.1 Percentage of patients over 60 years with infective endocarditis 1923-84 (adapted from Gantz[3]).

seems likely to continue as the numbers of old people continue to rise[4,5]. The male-to-female ratio is of the order of 1.5–2.0:1, though some series in the elderly have found higher proportions of males[6,7]. The reasons for this male preponderance are as yet unexplained. However, possible reasons are the decreasing numbers of rheumatic heart disease which predominated in females and the incidence of calcified and bicuspid aortic valves which is higher in males.

The mortality rate in the years after Osler's classic description of 'malignant endocarditis' in 1885, but before the advent of sulphonamides and penicillin in the 1940s, was virtually 100% and was due almost entirely to uncontrolled infection. Antibiotics reduced this to 30–40%[8] and most deaths are now due to secondary factors such as heart failure. This mortality rate has remained unaltered over the last 30 years [7,9,10] despite more powerful antibiotics, improved culture techniques and advances in intensive therapy. However, more recent studies indicate that the true mortality is nearer 15%[4,5,11]. A worse prognosis is found in most series for patients over 70 years old, with mortality rates of 45–72%[12,13]. The reasons for this include delay in diagnosis and treatment, and the presence of other serious illness. However, more recent studies indicate improving survival rates in the elderly[5,14]. Death is now usually attributable to the secondary effects of the disease rather than uncontrolled infection. The major causes of death are shown in Table 4.7. Uncontrollable heart failure is undoubtedly the major cause and any degree of heart failure carries a poorer prognosis.

Table 4.7 Major causes of death in infective endocarditis

Uncontrolled heart failure
Myocardial infarction
Myocardial involvement in infection
Arterial embolization
Mycotic aneurysm
Renal dysfunction

Predisposing Factors

The predisposing factors are an abnormality of a heart valve and a portal of entry for an infecting organism. The aortic valve is the site most commonly affected especially in the elderly. Both aortic and mitral valves are affected in 10–15% of cases[12, 14, 15]. These findings reflect the changing prevalence of degenerative and rheumatic heart diseases, the combination of congenital, degenerative and prosthetic valve endocarditis, together with cardiac surgery, have replaced rheumatic heart disease as the valvular lesion.

Unfortunately the portal of entry of the infection may be difficult to identify[5]. However, dental procedures still account for a minority of cases of endocarditis, despite the use of prophylactic antibiotics. Abnormalities and surgery of the gastrointestinal tract account for some cases of enterococcal endocarditis as does instrumentation of the genitourinary tract ('catheter fever'). In the elderly, decubitus ulcers and compound fractures are portals of entry that are often forgotten. Other predisposing factors are shown in Table 4.8.

Table 4.8 Factors influencing the development of endocarditis

Predisposing diseases and therapies
Congenital and degenerative heart disease
Rheumatic heart disease
Prosthetic valves
Hypertrophic subaortic stenosis
Previous infective endocarditis
Diabetes
Alcohol-related diseases
Immunosuppressive therapy
Renal failure
Malignant diseases

Portals of entry

Procedures or operations	dental urogenital alimentary
Infections or malignancies	urogenital alimentary skin
Fractures	
Intravenous lines	
Prosthetic implants	pacemakers and orthopaedic prostheses

Microbiology

The micro-organisms causing endocarditis are similar in the elderly and younger age groups with streptococci and staphylococci causing over two-thirds of cases. *Coxiella burnetti, Haemophilus influenza, Escherichia coli* and fungal infections account for proportionately fewer cases. The sharp increase in Gram-negative septicaemia in the elderly has not been mirrored by a similar rise in Gram-negative endocarditis[5, 12].

Among the streptococci, *S. viridans* is still the most common causative agent. However enterococci such as *S. faecalis* and *S. bovis* account for more cases in the elderly than in the younger age group. Alimentary surgery or intrumentation is a common portal of entry for *S. faecalis*[16], and the finding of *S. bovis* raises the possibility of colorectal carcinoma.

Staphylococcal endocarditis has a higher mortality rate overall and is particularly involved in prosthetic valve endocarditis (PVE). More people are surviving to the older age group with prosthetic valves and this may become an increasing problem in the future. PVE may be either early or late and occurs in about 1% of prosthetic valve implants. Early PVE that occurs within 2 months of operation is due largely to staphylococci, Gram-negative bacilli or fungi, *Candida albicans* and aspergillus. Late PVE still has a predominance of staphylococcal infections but *S. viridans* also causes 25% and it also has a lower mortality than early PVE[5, 8]. Most series include 10–15% of culture-negative endocarditis and failure to demonstrate a pathogen can be due to recent antibiotic administration, fastidious organisms or non-infective endocarditis.

Pathology and Pathogenesis

The characteristic valvular lesion in infective endocarditis is the vegetation. These vary in size from 1 mm to several millimetres in diameter, and are usually found on the downstream side of a high pressure lesion, that is, on the ventricular surface of the aortic valve, the atrial surface of the mitral valve and the right heart side of a ventricular septal defect. Animal studies have shown that in order for endocarditis to develop, the endocardial (valve) surface must be damaged in some way. In humans this damage may be due to the effects of a high pressure jet on, for example, the left atrial wall near the mitral valve. Once damage has occurred platelets and fibrin are deposited and these form a site for bacterial growth. *S. viridans* has been shown to have a particular affinity for these sites and thus may be accounted for by its morphological shape[17]. However this model does not account for the apparent absence of predisposing cardiac lesion in 30% of patients[5, 8]. Even when the valves of cases of infective endocarditis are examined pathologically, no underlying lesion is found in 30%[15].

Local spread of infection into surrounding tissues can lead to myocardial infarction, conduction abnormalities and arrhythmias, and purulent pericarditis. Acute or chronic destruction of the valve can lead to heart failure, and embolization can occur to any organ, particularly the brain and coronary arteries.

Embolization to the brain can lead to meningitis, cerebral abscess or mycotic aneurysm. Other non-cardiac manifestations of infective endocarditis are legion, and are caused either by microembolization or immunological phenomena, though it can be difficult to distinguish between the two.

Immunological mechanisms are implicated in some clinical features. Immune complexes can be identified in cutaneous and renal lesions and stainable immunoglobulins have been found in vessels in the skin and kidneys[18, 19]. High levels of circulating immune complexes have also been found to correlate with the development of renal lesions and vasculitic skin lesions. It has been suggested that circulating immune complexes may be a marker of infective endocarditis and also of the efficacy of treatment[20]. There was, however, no correlation with mucosal haemorrhage, Osler's nodes or Janeway lesions, inferring that these were microembolic phenomena. Musculoskeletal manifestations occur in 20% of cases of infective endocarditis, and though they correlate with renal manifestations, it is not clear whether they are septic or immunological in origin[21].

Clinical Features

Infective endocarditis has protean manifestations and can present subtly at any age. However, in the elderly it can present atypically in up to 30% of cases with such symptoms as malaise, weight loss, anorexia and mental confusion. Fever may be absent in 5–10% of cases even after hospital admission, and this may be due to prior antibiotic administration or inability to mount a febrile response. This can occur in any infection in the elderly and is ill understood.

Diagnosis in the elderly may also be delayed because symptoms and signs are attributed to other diseases. This delay in diagnosis can lead to heart failure and valve rupture with a consequent increase in mortality. Back and joint pains may be attributed to arthritis or old age and neurological symptoms and signs such as hemiplegia, aphasia and confusion to more common causes of cerebrovascular disease. In 25% of elderly people, heart murmurs may be absent or attributed to other causes such as anaemia. Indeed the only manifestations of infective endocarditis in the elderly may be malaise and heart failure[8]. These problems in diagnosis probably account for the rate of up to 50% of missed diagnosis[12, 13, 15]. These features which differ in the elderly are shown in Table 4.9.

Table 4.9   Manifestations of infective endocarditis differing in the elderly

---

More common in the elderly

Congestive heart failure
Neurological signs, such as stroke, aphasia
Musculoskeletal symptoms and signs, such as backache

Less common in the elderly

Fever
Heart murmurs
Splenomegaly
Cutaneous manifestations, such as Roth spots, Janeway lesions

---

Investigations

The blood culture is the most important single investigation. Three sets should be taken over a period of 3–4 hours and usually over 90% will be positive. If there is significant doubt about diagnosis, treatment can be delayed for 1–2 days while further blood cultures are obtained. Any elderly patient with an unexplained illness, with or without a heart murmur, should have blood cultures taken, particularly in the presence of heart failure or neurological signs. Close collaboration with a microbiologist is required at all stages particularly if the first blood cultures are negative but the clinical suspicion remains high. It will then be necessary to culture for fastidious and slow-growing organisms such as *Coxiella burnetti*. In these situations it is useful to carry out paired serological tests for chlamydia, rickettsia or fungi. However, 6–20% of cultures remain negative due to inadequate culture techniques, recent antibiotics or the development of L forms of bacteria[1, 8].

Other laboratory tests are less helpful. The ESR and white blood count are usually raised, though the white blood count less so than in younger patients[12, 14]. Tests of renal function are of limited value as a high urea is not uncommon in elderly people. However haematuria has been found in up to 90% of cases, though figures of 25–30% are more usual. This variation may relate to the duration of symptoms[4, 13]. Low levels of serum complement, positive rheumatoid factor, and circulating immune complexes may be found but as yet have no definite place in diagnosis or management.

Treatment

Antibiotics are the mainstay of treatment and should be started immediately after blood cultures have been taken when the suspicion of infective endocarditis is strong. Again close collaboration with the microbiologist is required to ensure optimum therapy. In all but the most uncomplicated cases, blind therapy should be started with benzylpenicillin and gentamicin in bolus doses given intravenously. If staphylococcal endocarditis is suspected or if the patient is severely ill, then cloxacillin or flucloxacillin should be added. Once bacteriological confirmation is obtained the regimes given in Table 4.10 should be followed. A regime for culture-negative endocarditis is also included. Antibiotics should be given intravenously for 4–6 weeks, although uncomplicated natural valve *S. viridans* infections may be changed to oral amoxycillin for 2–4 weeks, after initial intravenous therapy.

The duration of therapy is still controversial but relapse rates with short 2-week courses seems to be significantly higher[22, 23]. Blood levels of drugs should be taken at intervals to ensure adequate serum concentrations and minimize side-effects, especially when using aminoglycosides.

Table 4.10 Antibiotic treatment of infective endocarditis

Organism	Antibiotic
S. viridans	benzylpenicillin
S. bovis	
S. faecalis	benzylpenicillin and
Other streptococci	gentamicin
Staphylococci	flucloxacillin or cloxacillin and gentamicin and benzylpenicillin
Prosthetic valve endocarditis	cloxacillin or flucloxacillin and gentamicin and benzylpenicillin
Culture negative endocarditis	benzylpenicillin and gentamicin

Management

It is essential to monitor the patient for changing murmurs and clinical evidence of heart failure or embolization. Infection at the portal of entry should be eliminated if possible.

Echocardiography can be helpful in diagnosis and management. Vegetations larger than 2mm or more can be identified on echocardiogram although thickened or heavily calcified valves can make this difficult. While by no means diagnostic, the echocardiogram may be a useful adjunct to other tests. Echocardiography may also be used in management for:

1. Early detection of aortic and mitral valve incompetence and failing left ventricular function. This may be detected echocardiographically before any clinical signs develop.

2. Detection of myocardial abscesses and large vegetations that predispose to embolization. Used serially, once or twice a week, the

echocardiogram can be useful in deciding when surgical intervention is necessary[24, 25].

Indications for Surgery

The role of surgery in infective endocarditis has become clearer in recent years. With increasing technical skills, the mortality rates for a combined medical and surgical approach are improving. The indications for possible surgical intervention are shown in Table 4.11. Congestive heart failure is the commonest cause of death in infective endocarditis[24] and early surgical intervention can decrease mortality in those with heart failure from 50% to 20% depending on the severity of heart failure at the time of operation.

Table 4.11 Indications for cardiac surgery in infective endocarditis

Moderate to severe heart failure
Uncontrolled infection
Staphylococcal and fungal infections
Recurrent systemic emboli
Prosthetic valve endocarditis
Suppurative pericarditis

Uncontrolled infection and repeated embolization are also indications for surgery and operation on infected valves is now routine, with little post-operative infection. Staphylococcal infections may be managed medically, but there is some evidence that these patients should have valve replacements regardless of their haemodynamic status[11, 26]. Purulent pericarditis will require surgical drainage. The possibility of surgical treatment means that complicated cases of infectious endocarditis should be managed within easy reach of a cardiac surgery unit as operation may have to be performed urgently. This should apply as much to the elderly as to younger patients if mortality rates are to be improved. To ensure that treatment has been adequate, patients should have repeat blood cultures and clinical reassessment at monthly intervals for 3 months after treatment has been completed.

Prophylaxis

The role of prophylaxis is blurred due to the percentage of the population undergoing dental procedures and invasive investigations, the lack of direct evidence that prophylactic treatment is effective and the large proportion (40%) of cases of infective endocarditis who have either normal hearts or unrecognized heart lesions at the time of dental procedures. Moreover, evidence from the British Cardiac Society and Royal College of Physicians

Working Party[1, 5, 16] also suggests that antibiotic prophylaxis should seriously be considered for any genitourinary or alimentary procedure, especially in the elderly. When prophylaxis is to be used, the recommendations of the American Heart Association in 1977[27] are unpractical. A much more practical approach was offered by the British Society for Antimicrobial Therapy in 1982[28] and this is summarized in Table 4.12. Table 4.13 lists the procedures for which prophylaxis is recommended and those for which it should be seriously considered, especially in those with an underlying heart lesion, or other conditions such as malignancy, diabetes and immunosupression which could lead to decreased resistance to infecting organisms in individual patients. It should be borne in mind that occasional failures of even the most up-to-date prophylaxis have been reported[29]. Finally it may be that all elderly people should be considered for prophylaxis as they appear to have an increased risk, and normal hearts also appear to be vulnerable[5].

Table 4.12 Antibiotic prophylaxis

Dental procedures	amoxycillin 3g orally 1 hour before procedure
If allergic to penicillin or have had penicillin recently	erythromycin 1.5g 2 hours before procedure; erythromycin 0.5g 6 hours after procedure
Dental procedure with general anaesthetic	amoxycillin 1g and local anaesthetic intramuscularly before induction; amoxycillin 0.5g orally 6 hours after; patients allergic to penicillin or with prosthetic valves should be referred to hospital
Other procedures or operations	amoxycillin 1g (with local anaesthetic) and gentamicin 120mg immediately before procedure or induction of anaesthetic; vancomycin should be used in penicillin-sensitive patients

Table 4.13 Antibiotic prophylaxis procedures

Recommended in patients with known heart lesions

All dental procedures
Genitourinary procedures or operations

Considered in patients with known heart lesions

Gastroscopy
Colonoscopy
Alimentary surgery including herniorrhaphy
Gynaecological surgery
Compound fractures

References to Part I: Septicaemia

1. Powrie, S. and Norman J. (1976). Septicaemia. *Br. J. Anaesth.*, **48,** 41–7
2.. Watt, P. J. and Okubadejo, O. A. (1967). Changes in the incidence and aetiology of bacteraemia arising in hospital practice. *Br. Med. J.*, **1,** 210–11
3. Crowley, N. (1970). Some bacteraemia encountered in hospital practice. *J. Clin. Pathol.*, **23,** 166–71
4. McGowan, J. E., Barnes, M. W. and Finland, M. (1975). Bacteraemia at Boston General Hospital. *J. Infect. Dis.*, **132,** 316–35
5. McHenry, D. C., Martin, W. J. and Wellman, W. E. (1962). Bacteraemia due to Gram-negative bacilli. *Ann. Intern. Med.*, **56,** 207–19
6. Weil, M. H. and Shubin, H. (1973). Treatment of shock caused by bacterial infections. *West. J. Med.*, **119,** 7–13
7. Jepson, O. B. and Korner, B. (1975). Bacteraemia in a general hospital. *Scand. J. Infect. Dis.*, **7,** 179–83
8. Windsor, A. C. M. (1983). Bacteraemia in a geriatric unit. *Gerontology*, **29,** 125–30
9. Faber, V., Jessen, O., Rosendal, K. and Erikson, K. R. (1960). Staphylococcal bacteraemia. *Br. Med. J.*, **2,** 1832–6
10. Altmeier, W. A., Todd, J. C. and Inge, W. W. (1967). Gram-negative septicaemia: a growing threat. *Ann. Surg.*, **166,** 530–42
11. Jansson, E. (1971). A 10 year study of bacteraemia. *Scand. J. Infect. Dis.*, **3,** 151–5
12. Kreger, B. E., Croven, D. E. and McCabe, W. R. (1980). Gram-negative bacteraemia (III): Reassessment of aetiology, epidemiology and ecology in 612 patients. *Am. J. Med.*, **68,** 332–43
13. Madden, J. W., Croher, J. R. and Beynon, G. P. J. (1981). Septicaemia in the elderly. *Postgrad. Med. J.*, **57,** 502–6
14. Finland, M., Jones, W. F. and Barnes, M. W. (1959). Occurrence of serious bacterial infections since the introduction of antibiotics. *J. Am. Med. Assoc.*, **170,** 2188–97
15. Kreger, B. E., Craven, D. E. and McCabe, W. R. (1980). Gram-negative bacteraemia (IV) Re-evaluation of clinical features and treatment in 612 patients. *Am. J. Med.*, **168,** 344–55
16. Winslow, E. J., Loeb, H., Rabinkoola, S. H., Kamath, S. and Gunnar, R. M. (1973). Haemodynamic studies and the results of therapy in 50 patients with bacteraemic shock. *Am. J. Med.*, **54,** 421–32
17. Esposito, A. L., Gleckman, R. A., Cram, S., Crowley, M., McCabe, F. and Drapkin, M. S. (1980). Community acquired bacteraemia in the elderly; analysis of one hundred consecutive episodes. *J. Am. Geriat. Soc.*, **28,** 315–19
18. Fein, A. M., Lippman, M., Holtzman, H., Eliraz, A. and Goldberg, S. K. (1983). The risk factors incidence and prognosis of ARDS following septicaemia. *Chest*, **83,** 40–2
19. Le Froch, J., Ellis, C. A., Turclik, J. B. and Weinstein, L. (1973). Transient bacteraemia associated with sigmoidoscopy. *N. Engl. J. Med.*, **289,** 467–9
20. McClosky, R. V., Gold, M. and Weser, E. (1973). Bacteraemia after liver biopsy. *Arch. Intern. Med.*, **132,** 213–5
21. Pelican, G., Hentages, D., Butt, J., Haag, J., Holfer, R. and Hutcheson D. (1976). Bacteraemia during colonoscopy. *Gastrointest. Endoscopy*, **23,** 33–5
22. Hoffman, B. I., Kobasa, W. and Kaage, D. (1978). Bacteraemia after rectal examination. *Ann. Intern. Med.*, **88,** 658–9
23. Camara, D. S., Graber, M., Barde, C. J., Moules, M., Caruana, J. A. and Chung, R. S. (1983). Transient bacteraemia following endosopic injection sclerotherapy of esophageal varices. *Arch. Intern. Med.*, **143,** 1350–2
24. Br. Med. J. (1975). Editorial: Bacteraemia from the bowel. **21,** 396–7
2,5. Denham, M. J. and Goodwin, C. S. (1977). The value of blood cultures in geriatric practice. *Age Ageing*, **6,** 85–8
26. Svanbom, M. (1979). Septicaemia I: A prospective study of aetiology, underlying factors and sources of infection. *Scand. J. Infect. Dis.*, **12,** 189–206
27. Klein, R. S., Catalano, M. T., Edberg, S. C., Casey, J. I. and Steigbigel, N. H. (1979). *Streptococcus bovis* septicaemia and carcinoma of the colon. *Ann. Intern. Med.*, **91,** 560–562
28. McGovern, V. J. (1972). The pathophysiology of Gram-negative septicaemia. *Pathology*, **4,** 265–71

29. Cooper T. J. and Tinker, J. (1984). The adult respiratory distress syndrome. *Hosp. Update*, **10**, 849–59
30. Hurewitz, A. and Bergofsky, E. H. (1981). Adult respiratory distress syndrome. Physiological basis for treatment. *Med. Clin. N. Am.*, **65 (1)**, 33–51
31. Wardle, N. (1979). Bacteraemia and endotoxic shock. *Br. J. Hosp. Med.*, **21**, 223–31
32. Dietzmann, R. H. and Lillehein, R. C. (1968). The nature and treatment of shock. *Br. J. Hosp. Med.*, **1**, 300–304
33. McCabe, W. R., Treadwell, T. L. and DeMaria, A. (1983). Pathophysiology of bacteraemia. *Am. J. Med.*, **75 (1B)**, 7–18
34. Rheingold, A. L., Horgreth, N. T., Dan, B. B. B., Shands, K. N., Strickland, B. Y. and Broome, C. V. (1982). Non-menstrual toxic shock syndrome. *Ann. Intern. Med.*, **96 (2)**, 871–4
35. Chow, W. C., Wong, C. K., Goldring MacFarlane, A. M. and Barlett, K. H. (1983). Toxic shock syndrome. Clinical and laboratory findings in 30 patients. *Can. Med. Assoc. J.*, **130**, 425–30
36. Shands, K. N. *et al.* (1980). Toxic shock syndrome in menstruating women. Association with tampon use and *Staphylococcus aureus*, and clinical features in 52 cases. *N. Engl. J. Med.*, **303**, 1436–42
37. Tofte, R. W. and Williams, D. N. (1981). Toxic shock syndrome. Clinical and laboratory features in 15 patients. *Ann. Intern. Med.*, **94**, 149–56
38. Paris, A. L., Herwaldt, L. A., Blum, D., Shmidt, P. G., Shands, K. N. and Broome, C. V. (1981). Pathological findings in twelve fatal cases of toxic shock syndrome. *Ann. Intern. Med.*, **96 (2)**, 852–7
39. Jones, P. G., Kauffman, C. A., Bergman, A. G., Hayes, C. M., Kluger, M. J. and Cannon, J. G. (1984). Fever in the elderly: production of leukocyte pyrogen by monocytes from elderly persons. *Gerontology*, **30**, 182–7
40. Lees, N. W. (1976). The diagnosis and treatment of endotoxic shock. *Anaesthesia*, **31**, 897–904
41. McLean, L. D., Mulligan, W. G., McLean, A. P. H. and Daff, J. H. (1967). Patterns of septic shock in man – a detailed study of 56 patients. *Ann. Surg.*, **166**, 543–62
42. Emmanouel, D. S. and Katz, A. K. (1973). Acute renal failure in obstetric septic shock. *Am. J. Obstet. Gynecol.*, **117**, 145–9
43. Morrison, D. C. and Cochrane, C. G. (1974). Direct evidence for Hagemann factor (Factor XII) activation by bacterial lipopolysaccharides (endotoxins). *J. Exp. Med.*, **140**, 797–811
44. Colman, R. W., Robhem, S. J. and Minna, J. P. (1972). Disseminated intravascular coagulation (DIC): an approach. *Am. J. Med.*, **52**, 679–689
45. Finkelstein, M. S., Petkun, W. M., Freedman, M. L. and Antopol, S. C. (1983). Pneumococcal bacteraemia in adults: age dependent differences in presentation and outcome. *J. Am. Geriatr. Soc.*, **31**, 19–27
46. Inglis, T. J. J. and Millar, M. R. (1984). Diminished response to endotoxin. *Br. Med. J.*, **289**, 734
47. Centre for Disease Control (1974). Contamination of blood culture medium. *Kentucky, Maryland Morbid Mortal Week. Rep.*, **23 (12)**, 109–110
48. Kaslow, R. A., Machel, D. C. and Mallinson, G. F. (1976). Nosocomial pseudobacteraemia; positive blood cultures due to a contaminated benzalkonium antiseptic. *J. Am. Med. Assoc.*, **236**, 2407–8
49. Berkelman, R. C., Lewin, S. and Allen, J. R. (1981). Pseudobacteraemia attributed to contamination of povidone-iodine with *Pseudomonas cepacia*. *Ann. Intern. Med.*, **95**, 32–6
50. McLowry, J. D. (1983). Clinical microbiology of bacteraemia: an overview. *Am. J. Med.*, **28**, 2–6
51. Geddes, A. M. (1978). Use of antibiotics: septicaemia. *Br. Med. J.*, **2**, 181–4
52. Elin, R. J., Robinson, R. A., Levine, A. S. *et al.* (1975). Lack of clinical usefulness of the Limulus test in the diagnosis of endotoxaemia. *N. Engl. J. Med.*, **293**, 521–4
53. Reik, H. and Rubin, S. J. (1981). Evaluation of the buffy coat smear for the rapid detection of bacteraemia. *J. Am. Med. Assoc.*, **245**, 357–9
54. Lynch, J. M., Hodges, G. R., Clark, G. M. and Dworzach, D. C. (1981). Gram-negative bacteraemias: analysis of factors for clinical assessment of gentamicin resistance. *Arch. Intern. Med.*, **141**, 582–6

55. Ledingham, I. McA. and McArdle, C. S. (1978). Prospective study of the treatment of septic shock. *Lancet*, **1,** 1194–7
56. Collier, J. G., Herman, A. G. and Vane, J. R. (1973). Appearance of prostaglandins in the renal venous blood of dogs in response to acute systemic hypotension produced by bleeding or endotoxin. *J. Physiol.*, **230,** 19
57. Fletcher, J. R. (1982). The role of prostaglandins in sepsis. *Scand. J. Infect. Dis.*, Suppl. 31, 55–60
58. Zeigler, E. J., McCutchon, J. A., Fhirer, J., Glauser, M. P., Sadoff, J. C., Douglas, H. and Brande, A. I. (1982). Treatment of Gram-negative bacteraemia and shock with human antiserum to a mutant *Escherichia coli*. *N. Engl. J. Med.*, **20,** 1225–30

References to Part II: Infective Endocarditis

1. Bayliss, R., Clarke, C., Oakley, C. M., Somerville W. and Whitfield, A. G. W. (1983). The teeth and endocarditis. *Br. Heart J.*, **50,** 506–12
2. Kelson, S. R. and White, P. D. (1945). Notes on 250 cases of subacute bacterial (streptococcal) endocarditis studied and treated between 1927 and 1939. *Ann. Intern. Med.*, **22,** 40
3. Gantz, N. M. (1983). Infective endocarditis. In Gleckman, R. A. and Gantz, N. M. (eds.) *Infections in the elderly* (Boston: Little and Brown)
4. Von Reyn, C. F., Levy, B. S., Arbeit, R. D. *et al.* (1981). Infective endocarditis. An analysis based on strict case definitions.
5. Bayliss, R., Clarke, C., Oakley, C. M., Somerville, W., Whitfield, A. G. W. and Young, S. E. J. (1983). The microbiology and pathogenesis of infective endocarditis. *Br. Med. J.*, **50,** 513–19
6. Rabbinovich, S., Evans, J., Smith, I. O. M. and January, L. E. (1965). A long term view of bacterial endocarditis: 337 cases 1924–1963. *Ann. Intern. Med.*, **63,** 185
7. Lerner, P. O. and Weinstein, L. (1966). Infective endocarditis in the antibiotic era. *N. Engl. J. Med.*, **274,** 199
8. Cantrell, M. and Yoshikawa, T. T. (1983). Ageing and infective endocarditis. *J. Am. Geriatr. Soc.*, **31,** 216–22
9. Smith, R. H., Radford, D. J., Clark, R. A. and Julian, D. G. (1976). Infective endocarditis in the South East Region of Scotland. 1967–1972, *Thorax*, **31,** 373–9
10. Garvey, G. J. and Neu, H. F. (1978). Infective endocarditis, an evolving disease. *Medicine*, **57,** 105–27
11. Richardson, J. V., Karp, R. B., Kirklin, J. W. and Dismukes, W. E. (1978). Treatment of infective endocarditis: a 10-year comparative analysis. *Circulation*, **54,** 584–597
12. Robbins, N., Demania, A. and Miller, M. H. (1980). Infective endocarditis in the elderly. *S. Med. J.*, **73,** 1335
13. Applefield, M. M. and Hornick, R. B. (1974). Infective endocarditis in patients over age 60. *Am. Heart J.*, **88,** 90
14. Tan, J. S., Watanakunakern, C. and Terherne, C. A. Jr. (1973). *Streptococcus viridans* endocarditis: favorable prognosis in geriatric patients. *Geriatrics*, **28,** 68
15. Thell, R., Martin, E. H. and Edwards, J. E. (1975). Bacterial endocarditis in Sahjeds 60 years of age and older. *Circulation*, **51,** 174–82
16. Bayliss, R., Clarke, C., Oakley, C., Somerville, W., Whitfield, A. G. W. and Young, S. E. J. (1984). The bowel, the genitourinary tract and infective endocarditis. *Br. Heart J.*, **51,** 339–45
17. *Brit. Med. J.* (1975). Editorial. Bacteraemia from the bowel, **2,** 396–7
18. Harmer, J. and O'Grady, F. (1977). In: Harmer, J. (ed) *Advance in Cardiology*. Vol 4, p.447. (Edinburgh: Churchill Livingstone)
19. Lowenstein, M. B., Vrman, J. D., Aboley, M. and Weistein, A. (1977). Skin immunofluorescence in infective endocarditis. *J. Am. Med. Assoc.*, **238,** 1163–5

20. Kauffman, R. H., Thompson, J., Valeentign, R. M., Mohammed, M. R. and Van Es, L. A. (1981). The clinical implications and pathogenetic significance of circulating immune complexes in infective endocarditis. *Am. J. Med.*, **71,** 17–25

21. Thomas, J., Allal, D., Bontoux, F., Rossi, F., Poupet, Y., Petitalot, J. P. and Becq-Giradedon, B. (1984). Rheumatological manifestations of infective endocarditis. *Ann. Rheum. Dis.*, **43,** 716–20

22. Oakley, C. M. (1980). Infective endocarditis. *Br. J. Hosp. Med.*, **2,** 232–43

23. Hanson, D. C. (1983). Prophylaxis and treatment of infectious endocarditis: current recommendations. *Drugs,* **25,** 433–9

24. Brandenburg, R. O., Giuliani, E. R., Wilson, W. R. and Geraci, J. E. (1983). Infective endocarditis. A 25 year overview of diagnosis and therapy. *J. Am. Coll. Cardiol.* **1,** 280–91

25. Mann, T., McLaurin, L., Grossman, W. and Craig, E. (1975). Assessing the haemodynamic severity of acute aortic regurgitation due to infective endocarditis. *N. Engl. J. Med.*, **293,** 108–113

26. Perry, L. S., Tresch, D. A., Brooks, H. L., Lepley, D., Olinger, G. N., Banchek, L. L. and Johnson, G. (1984). Operative approach to endocarditis. *Am. Heart J.*, **108** (11), 561–6

27. American Heart Association (1977). Prevention of bacterial endocarditis. *Circulation,* **56,** 139A–143A

28. British Society of Antimicrobial Therapy (1982). The antibiotic prophylaxis of infective endocarditis. *Lancet,* **2,** 1323–6

29. Denning, D. W., Casidy, M., Dougall, A. and Stewart Hilles, W. (1984). Failure of single dose amoxycillin as prophylaxis against endocarditis. *Br. Med. J.,* **289,** 1499–1500

5

Infective Diarrhoea

H. SMITH

INTRODUCTION

Although the similarities outweigh the differences between gastrointestinal infections in the aged, and in the general adult population, there are, nevertheless, sufficient differences in presentation, incidence, epidemiology and pathology to warrant separate consideration for infective diarrhoea in old age. This chapter deals with gastrointestinal infections in general, emphasizing the particular problems of the aged, and examines some common contemporary problems.

PRESENTATION

At the outset it must be emphasized that the term infective diarrhoea implies an accepted aetiology, and that in the vast majority of patients the clinical presentation will be with diarrhoea, diarrhoea and vomiting, 'gastroenteritis' or some such non-specific tag. It cannot be too strongly stated that these non-specific gastrointestinal symptoms can be caused by a whole range of disorders which are not primarily of infective origin; inflammatory bowel disease, neoplasms, metabolic disorders such as diabetic acidosis, intestinal obstruction, and peritonitis in all its variations are a few examples of the many conditions which may be confused with gastrointestinal infections. These caveats apply in all age groups but particularly to older patients who probably have more frequent episodes of infective diarrhoea as a result of the reduction in gastric acid which accompanies increasing age, and also because geriatric patients are more likely to have existing bowel pathology simply because of their age. Thus infection may complicate known or presumed intestinal disorders. Patients who are infirm, confined to bed, often being treated for chronic illness, may have poor muscle tone, become constipated and develop what amounts to secondary megacolon. Large collections of faeces may present clinically as multiple small stools, what is essentially faecal incontinence due to a lax sphincter. In chronically ill patients this is a frequent mode of presentation; rectal examination provides the diagnosis and often the cure.

EPIDEMIOLOGY

Infective diarrhoea is extremely common; in developing countries it presents major public health problems and life-threatening illness is common in the young. Enteritis and other diarrhoeal disease was classified by the World Health Organization in 1974 as amongst the ten leading causes of death. In industrially developed countries gastrointestinal infections are less common but are responsible for much lost production, morbidity, discomfort and occasional deaths, especially at the extremes of life.

If we take the total number of notifications of gastrointestinal infections to the Communicable Disease Surveillance Centre (CDSC) at Colindale as an indication of the general prevalence of these infections in the United Kingdom we note a slight rise during the period 1979–1983. Campylobacter accounted for more reported infections than salmonellae; the total number of salmonella infections notified for 1983 (14325) was greater than in any of the last 20 years (range 3898 in 1966 to 12218 in 1979). Shigella infections also increased in number and this is probably accounted for by large outbreaks of Sonne dysentry in the north of England. These trends continued in 1984.

Introduction of new techniques have probably been responsible for some of the increase in notification of rotavirus infection. Since 1978 approximately 6% of reports have involved rotavirus infection in children under 4, but there has been an increase (0.5–1.3%) in the number of notifications in those aged 65 or over.

In enterocolitis due to *Clostridium difficile* – one of the forms of antibiotic associated diarrhoea – there would seem to be a much higher incidence in older age groups. As *Cl. difficile* enterocolitis is not notifiable, no precise figures are available, but in many institutions and hospitals the geriatric population seems to be at increased risk.

Many general statements on epidemiology are unhelpful or are irrelevant when faced with a number of possibly related cases of diarrhoea in an individual hospital or ward. Undoubtedly the local situation is of much greater importance than the overall incidence of particular forms of infective diarrhoea.

PATHOPHYSIOLOGY OF DIARRHOEA

About 8 l of fluid enters the duodenum each day and, allowing for an average western man's diet, perhaps 200–300 ml is lost in the stool. Absorption of this large volume of fluid appears to be entirely a function of osmotic pressure gradients; there is no evidence for a specific metabolic process as the intestinal mucosa acts as a semipermeable membrane with varying degrees of permeability throughout its length. Most evidence now suggests that absorption of water in the intestine occurs between rather than through the epithelial cells. Absorption of water and electrolytes is to some extent controlled or modified by a variety of hormones and polypeptides; from the point of view of infective diarrhoea the most important of these is the cyclic AMP adenyl cyclase system which is implicated in the secretory diarrhoea induced by cholera toxin; some strains of *E. coli* and perhaps other bacteria also act via the cyclic AMP pathway.

MICROBIOLOGY OF NORMAL GUT FLORA

The indigenous bacterial flora of the gut exerts an extraordinary stabilizing effect, which can be considered a normostatic mechanism. In terms of relative populations of different organisms, as well as the elaboration of a number of metabolites – lactic acid, short-chain fatty acids – the microflora represents a major protection against infection and consequently protects against diarrhoea. Derangement of these homeostatic mechanisms, as in bacterial overgrowth due to blind loop syndromes or in the upsets that can result from antimicrobial drugs, may so alter bowel flora that diarrhoea is one of the inevitable results.

The oesophagus and stomach contain a relatively sparse flora of organisms derived from the oropharynx – often Gram-positive cocci, *Neisseria* species and *Haemophilus* strains – carried there in ingested food and liquid. Of major importance in coping with these bacteria is the gastric acid; an increase in pH allows many more oganisms to survive and to be carried further into the intestine. Increase in age, the use of antacids or H₂-antagonists, or gastric surgery can modify gastric acidity so that many more ingested organisms survive, and presumably multiply and cause severe symptoms.

Normally the upper duodenum has a sparse flora and the jejunum is in most cases sterile. A major change occurs at the ileocaecal valve where Gram-negative species are encountered so that the colon is literally teaming with *E. coli* and a whole range of anaerobes particularly *Bacteroides* species.

PATHOGENIC MECHANISMS OF DIARRHOEA

There are at least three ways in which micro-organisms can cause diarrhoea: by toxins, by cytotoxin formation, and by direct invasion.

Toxins

Adenyl cyclase catalyses the formation of cyclic AMP from ATP in the basolateral membrane of the intestinal villus epithelium. Cyclic AMP is responsible for secretion and stimulation of villous cyclic AMP which results in increased intraluminal secretion. This is the mechanism induced by cholera toxin. Jejunal biopsies obtained during the course of cholera show an increased concentration of cyclic AMP in the acute phase of the illness compared to the convalescent phase. Inhibition of enzymes responsible for the breakdown of cyclic AMP leads to increased concentrations and to increased secretion from the intestinal mucosa. Adenyl cyclase stimulation by cholera toxin seems to be an 'all or nothing' phenomenon so that recovery from cholera depends upon the replacement of affected cells by new ones migrating from the crypts to the villi.

Enterotoxins have been described in various strains of *E. coli* – at least two varieties exist, heat-stable toxin (ST) and heat-labile toxin (LT). Both these enterotoxins are capable of producing secretory diarrhoea – LT resembles cholera toxin physiologically and antigenically and would appear to cause diarrhoea in a manner closely resembling cholera toxin.

A heat-labile, non-dialysable toxin, neutralized by *Cl. sordelli* produced by *Cl. difficile,* has now been shown to be responsible for one of the major forms of antibiotic-induced diarrhoea – pseudomembranous enterocolitis.

At least five heat-stable enterotoxins are recognized in certain strains of *Staph. aureus* which are implicated in food-borne illness. Occasionally secretory disturbances and mucosal biochemical abnormality have been noted but the primary effect of staphylococcal enterotoxin appears to be on the medullary vomiting centre.

Cytotoxins

Instead of producing secretory diarrhoea induced by enterotoxin, a disturbance of the tip of the microvilli by locally acting cytotoxins has been demonstrated in a number of bacterial species. This has been most convincingly demonstrated in the case of *Cl. difficile,* but almost certainly similar cytotoxins are responsible for some of the pathogenic effects of some *Shigella* species and some strains of *E. coli.* In the latter species the cytotoxin strains produce diarrhoea independent of LT and ST and may relate to the adherent properties of these organisms.

Direct Invasion

Although *Shigella* species may produce enterotoxins and cytotoxins they represent the prime instance of organisms which produce their effects by tissue invasion. *Shigella* species differ in the proportion of disorder resulting from toxins or invasion. *Sh. dysenteriae* for instance, usually associated with a severe illness characterized by marked mucus and blood loss in the stools, produces its effect almost entirely by colonic disruption induced by bacterial invasion.

It is surprising to note that the disorder resulting from salmonella infection is far from being completely understood. In typhoid fever the inflammatory reaction in Peyer's patches and lymphoid follicles in the small bowel clearly relates to diarrhoea and the complications of haemorrhage and perforation of the bowel. In the much commoner salmonellosis – the food poisoning variety of salmonella infection – the pathogenesis is for the most part conjectural; toxins and prostaglandins may be implicated.

MANAGEMENT OF DIARRHOEA

General Aspects: Fluid Requirements

Most cases of infective gastrointestinal upset can be managed simply and do not demand specific medical care. If symptoms are severe, or prolonged, or both, the inevitable consequence is water deprivation, with or without electrolyte disturbance. At one extremity of the range of illness is cholera, which usually demands intravenous infusion to maintain adequate circulation and perfusion of vital tissues, while some patients who have been ill for days may be able to maintain adequate fluid intake via the oral route. In these patients a continued trial of oral fluids is often justified. Indications for intravenous therapy include increasing tachycardia, falling blood pressure, reduced urine flow, increased drowsiness as well as the common clinical indicators of dehydration. In assessing the clinical state care should be taken to know what drugs the patient may have been taking before the onset of gastrointestinal symptoms. Thus in older patients who are frequently receiving beta-blocking agents, oligaemia may not produce the expected tachycardia and a dangerous degree of hypotension may result. In general, water containing a low concentration of electrolytes (as in Dioralyte or half-strength Hartmann's solution) is the safest to administer until serum electrolyte values are available.

If there is clear evidence of hypokalaemia this should be corrected by potassium supplements. In general, once the circulatory volume has been restored, stable blood pressure and adequate urine flow maintained, the serum electrolyte concentrations take care of themselves as long as renal function is normal or near normal.

Relief of Symptoms: Antidiarrhoeal Compounds

Nearly all compounds used as antidiarrhoeal agents should be viewed with circumspection if not suspicion; if in fact they do prove effective, their action may not always be beneficial to the patient, for side-effects may dominate.

These drugs may be classified into four main groups: (1) antimuscarines, (2) opium alkaloids, (3) synthetic opium alkaloids, and (4) absorbents.

Antimuscarines

These are alkaloids of the belladonna plants which antagonize the muscarinic actions of acetylcholine. These include reduction in volume of salivary and gastric secretion and decrease in tone, amplitude and frequency in peristaltic action. Side-effects of dry mouth and blurred vision are common with therapeutic doses. A preparation such as Buscopan, (hyocine butylbromide 10mg) can sometimes be useful in relief of abdominal colic.

Opium Alkaloids

These are probably best avoided in view of the possibility of dependency; the major exception is codeine phosphate, often used in conjunction with kaolin or chalk.

Synthetic Opium Alkaloids

Pethidine is a synthetic analgesic drug and the related diphenoxylate has a morphine-like action on the bowel. Lomotil combines diphenoxylate with a small dose of atropine. Toxicity can occur particularly in children and a dangerous 'toxic megacolon' type syndrome may be induced. There are reasons for believing, not entirely theoretically, that Lomotil can occasionally make symptoms more severe in shigellosis and salmonellosis.

Absorbents

Inert substances such as kaolin or the purified carbohydrate pectin may help to increase the consistency of stools. There are no controlled trials showing the effects of these absorbents. Methylcellulose which adds bulk to the stool has the advantage that it may be used in the management both of constipation and diarrhoea.

Agents Inhibiting Intestinal Secretion

Prostaglandins which increase mucosal adenyl cyclase may be responsible for diarrhoea in such conditions as the carcinoid syndrome, and medullary carcinoma of the thyroid. They may also be implicated in the diarrhoea resulting from infection caused by some strains of *E. coli* and even salmonellae. Aspirin and indomethacin inhibit prostaglandins and have at least a theoretical role in treating diarrhoea due to these agents.

Conclusion

Severe diarrhoea probably cannot be controlled unless the cause is dealt with; some of the above compounds can make the patient more comfortable without removal of the cause of diarrhoea. Time, and in a few instances specific therapy, will effect cure.

Specific Therapy

Diarrhoea is more often a reason for withdrawing antimicrobial chemotherapy than for administering it. There are a number of well-defined exceptions where chemotherapy is beneficial and a larger number of controversial situations where these drugs are used on the basis of personal judgement, even prejudice, rather than on the evidence of controlled trials and scientific fact. Details of chemotherapy are given in the section on individual infections; Table 5.1 is given as a guide.

CAMPYLOBACTER INFECTION

Campylobacter infection is now the commonest cause of bacterial infective enteritis in the United Kingdom. The presentation is usually an acute diarrhoeal illness; bacteraemia is a rare complication. There may be a history of contact with animals. Stools may contain mucus and blood, pain is perhaps more marked than in similar infections due to salmonellae and the incubation period may extend to 4 days. Because of the character of the abdominal pain these patients are prone to be referred to surgical departments.

Isolation is advisable.

Treatment

Treatment is symptomatic; erythromycin is given in severe or prolonged illness or in debilitated patients.

Table 5.1   Chemotherapy in gastrointestinal infections

Infection	Specific antimicrobial therapy	Comment
Salmonellosis (uncomplicated)	contraindicated	Patients with 'gut-confined' salmonella infection should not be given antimicrobials
Salmonellosis (complicated) Typhoid Fever	chloramphenicol co-trimoxazole ampicillin	complications include: continuing septicaemia, focal infection
Bacillary dysentery	rarely required except for *Sh. dysenteriae* infection	treat severe infections only: ampicillin/co-trimoxazole
E. coli infection	contraindicated	treat bloodstream infections and occasionally debilitated subjects
Staph. aureus (food poisoning) (enterocolitis)	contraindicated antistaphylococcal agents such as cloxacillin	rare today
Campylobacter	contraindicated	erythromycin if severe or focal infection
Giardiasis	metronidazole/mepacrine	
Cl. difficile enterocolitis	metronidazole/vancomycin	often settles without therapy
Rotavirus infection	none available	
Vibrio cholerae	tetracycline	
Entamoeba histolytica	metronidazole	

SALMONELLA INFECTIONS

There are more than 2000 different species of salmonellae; with the exception of *S. typhi* and *S. paratyphi* the illness produced by these organisms is characterized predominantly by diarrhoea, often with fever and vomiting. *S. cholerae-suis* – a rare pathogen – is an exception, producing prolonged fever, often without gastrointestinal features and with a propensity for abscess formation. In any salmonella infection, bloodstream invasion may occur and focal infection result.

Typhoid Fever

Salmonella typhi is an unusual salmonella in that it is pathogenic for humans only, unlike the majority of these organisms which have animal reservoirs, often causing major veterinary problems. The clinical presentation of typhoid is with fever, headache, malaise, and constipation rather than diarrhoea; diarrhoea is seldom encountered until the third week of illness. Splenomegaly, rose spots and constitutional upset indicate the generalized nature of the illness in which bloodstream invasion is expected within the first week. Blood culture, as well as stool, and perhaps urine culture are important diagnostic investigations. The leukocyte count is within the normal range or there is often leukopaenia with a relative lymphocytosis. The Widal reaction is seldom helpful.

Isolation is obligatory.

Treatment

Treatment is supportive, and specific therapy is chloramphenicol, cotrimoxazole or ampicillin.

Salmonellosis

Commonly this type of infection manifests within 18–24 hours of ingestion of contaminated food – often *meat,* sausages, or meat pies. Fever, abdominal pain and, in the initial stages, vomiting may be noted, but diarrhoea is the characteristic complaint often with blood and mucus. Many cases settle spontaneously even though the organisms can be cultured from the stool for prolonged periods. Occasionally blood cultures are positive.

Salmonella infection is a common cause of institutional outbreaks of infective diarrhoea. Recent examples of cases in psychogeriatric units indicate the difficulties in control of these infections which are often contributory causes of death when large numbers of older patients are involved.

Three groups of patients are particularly vulnerable to salmonella infections:

1. Patients with sickle cell disease, who when infected with salmonella have a marked propensity to develop osteomyelitis.
2. Neonates, who may have bloodstream invasion with consequent focal infection.
3. Subjects in whom there is reduction of gastric acidity allowing a high proportion of salmonellae to survive. Patients who have had gastrectomy, or have pernicious anaemia, those taking alkalis or H_2-antagonists must be considered at increased risk. This group should probably include many geriatric patients in whom there is hypochlorhydria.

The relative lack of acidity means that even a small number of ingested organisms can result in diarrhoea; in some instances very florid watery diarrhoea may persist for several weeks and almost always produces some degree of renal failure. Dialysis may be required.

Isolation is obligatory.

Treatment

Treatment is supportive and symptomatic. Only severe or complicated cases require chemotherapy; here the drug of choice is chloramphenicol, with alternatives co-trimoxazole or ampicillin.

DYSENTERY

Bacillary

This is caused by the genus shigella of which there are four species. Bacillary dysentery is a relatively common infection – the usual pathogens encountered in the United Kingdom are *Sh. sonnei* and *Sh. flexneri; boydii* infection is extremely rare and *Sh. dystenteriae* is occasionally encountered as an imported infection and causes severe and protracted diarrhoea.

Unlike salmonellae, which for the most part are required in large numbers to produce clinical illness, even a few shigellae can cause disease. Thus infection can be transformed by fomites or even by contaminated hands.

The incubation period is short – a few days – and is followed by abdominal discomfort, diarrhoea, classically with stools containing blood, mucus and many leukocytes. There is usually fever and occasionally some patients present initially with meningism – thought to be due to a neurotoxin produced by some strains of shigellae. Bloodstream invasion is quite rare. Reactive arthritis may be a troublesome sequal. Dehydration is the exception and most cases (except those due to *Sh. dysenteriae)* are self-limiting. Chemotherapy should be reserved for seriously ill, debilitated patients; ampicillin or co-trimoxazole are the agents most likely to be effective.

Isolation is obligatory.

Amoebic

Amoebic dysentery, although ubiquitous, is mostly a problem in developing tropical countries; cases occurring in the United Kingdom almost invariably have a history of foreign travel. A few indigenous cases are on record. The incubation period is often about 1 month, but it may be as short as 1 week and may stretch to a year. The onset of symptoms is gradual and the patient is rarely toxic; diarrhoea with mucus and sometimes blood in the stool is noted – faecal leukocytes are not a marked feature.

The majority of patients present as a chronic or subacute illness with bouts of diarrhoea and abdominal discomfort. In some patients diarrhoea of intestinal amoebiasis is overlooked and the patient presents with features of liver abscess, acutely, or more often chronically with weight loss, fever and anorexia. Pain, which can be pleuritic in nature situated in the right lower chest suggests diaphragmatic or pleural involvement; linear atelectasis at the right lung base on a plain chest film can suggest the true seat of disease below the diaphragm. Occasionally some cases present with a tumour-like abdominal mass – the so-called amoeboma.

Intestinal perforation and stricture are occasionally encountered. Diagnosis depends on identifying trophozoites of *Entamoeba histolytica* in stool samples; material obtained by sigmoidoscopy can be particularly useful, when typical shallow colonic ulcers can be seen.

A useful addition to diagnostic methods includes the fluorescent antibody test, which is nearly always positive in invasive amoebiasis.

Treatment

Metronidazole has simplified the treatment of amoebiasis. It is suitable for (1) intestinal amoebiasis, (2) amoebic liver abscess, (3) asymptomatic cyst excretors. The drug should be given for at least 10 days. Occasionally second courses are required. Chloroquine, hydroxyquinolone, or combined therapy with tetracycline are rarely used today. Ultrasound and computed tomographic imaging have simplified the diagnosis and management of hepatic abscess; aspiration, if required, can be carried out under radiological control.

E. COLI INFECTION

Strains of *E. coli* are most often encountered as a cause of diarrhoea in small outbreaks in infants, as a cause of 'travellers diarrhoea' and occasionally sporadically in adults.

STAPHYLOCOCCAL INFECTION

Staphylococcus aureus may occasionally produce an enterocolitis resulting from the rapid overgrowth of antibiotic-resistant organisms resulting in severe watery diarrhoea with stools containing many Gram-positive cocci and leukocytes. This appears to be an increasingly rare complication of antibiotic usage which was most often encountered in postoperative patients.

Enterotoxin-producing strains of *Staph. aureus* are a common cause of 'food poisoning' – the infected food often being of the cream bun or milk product type.

The illness results from the ingestion of preformed toxins and the major symptom is vomiting, coming on within 2–4 hours of ingestion of the toxin-containing food. Supportive treatment, including intravenous fluid replacement in severe cases is sufficient. Isolation is not necessary.

GIARDIASIS

Giardia lamblia, a flagellate protozoan most often acquired from contaminated drinking water, is responsible for the protracted, intermittent gastrointestinal symptoms referred to as giardiasis. Flatulence, foul-smelling stools and evidence of malabsorption may be noted. Weight loss is occasionally quite marked.

Identification of giardia in the stool is the usual method of diagnosis. Aspiration of small bowel is an alternative method of obtaining suitable samples; this can be achieved suitably by the 'string test'. The patient swallows a small dissolvable capsule containing a length of fine string one end of which is firmly taped to the area around the patient's mouth or chin. When the capsule is judged to have reached the small bowel it is left in position for several hours. Removal of the string provides a sample of small bowel contents which may be removed from the string, placed on a glass slide and is available for immediate microscopy.

Isolation is not required.

Treatment

Metronidazole and mepacrine are the agents of choice in giardiasis.

ANTIBIOTIC-ASSOCIATED DIARRHOEA

It is probable that alteration in the gut microflora resulting from the administration of antibiotics is the major factor in the pathogenesis of this form of diarrhoea. It is also probably the single most important mechanism responsible for staphylococcal enterocolitis, described above. It is the postulated mechanism in many instances of diarrhoea in which antimicrobial agents are thought to be implicated but in which a clear aetiology cannot be established. The position with regards to *Cl. difficile*-induced enterocolitis appears to be more complex.

Cl. difficile *Diarrhoea*

Clostridium difficile is an anaerobic, spore-forming bacillus which is occasionally found in the stool of normal subjects. In one survey of 318 subjects, without diarrhoea, *Cl. difficile* was isolated in 3.1%. It is present in large numbers, together with its toxin in many cases of antibiotic-induced diarrhoea, in the severe instances of which pseudomembranes are found in the lumen of the colon. This form of pseudomembranous colitis (PMC) is now one of the commonest causes of diarrhoea encountered in patients receiving antibiotics, and is encountered in patients with diarrhoea almost as frequently as *Campylobacter* spp. One of the reasons for this statement is explained by the fact that we now have suitable methods of proving (stool culture: presence of toxin) the aetiology.

This form of diarrhoea does seem to be an important cause of diarrhoea in geriatric patients (in contrast *Cl. difficile* is usually a commensal in babies); this may be because geriatric patients frequently receive antibiotics. This refers not only to the therapeutic use of antibiotics but also prophylactic usage. There are well-described cases occurring in surgical and orthopaedic wards when prophylactic chemotherapy induced pseudomembranous colitis. In many cases the condition appears to spread by the faecal–oral route but also perhaps even by air spread. Outbreaks have been described after the use of contaminated sigmoidoscopes. Whatever the precise method of spread, pseudomembranous colitis occurring in a general ward should be considered seriously, and it is not sufficient to accept a single case as an isolated example of antibiotic-induced diarrhoea.

Spread to other patients should be prevented by removal of infected patients to an isolation unit. There must also be a reappraisal of nursing techniques, bedpan sterilization facilities and antibiotic usage.

Relation of Pseudomembranous Colitis to Antibiotics

Enterocolitis may follow the administration of almost any antimicrobial agent. Ampicillin, amoxycillin and tetracycline seem particularly prone to produce diarrhoea, but this may merely reflect the fashion of antibiotic usage. The newer cephalosporins, for instance, seem just as likely to be at fault as any of the older β-lactam compounds.

Diarrhoea may come on within a few days of starting the drug; it may also be delayed 2 weeks or more after its cessation. Diarrhoea, with mucus, and in severe cases blood in the motions is characteristic, when pseudomembranes may be seen on sigmoidoscopy. The majority of patients settle spontaneously when the antibiotic is withdrawn, but some persist with severe symptoms and fever. Abdominal pain, and tenderness, especially along the descending colon, can be very difficult to distinguish from colonic perforation. Some cases behave like severe inflammatory bowel disease. The demonstration of *Cl. difficile* and or its toxin in stools from such patients becomes an emergency investigation and indicates a clear course of management.

Management of Pseudomembranous Colitis

In cases where the diagnosis is proved or strongly suspected the offending drug should be withdrawn; an alternative should be substituted if the patient's condition demands it. Dehydration, if present, should be corrected.

In severe persisting cases either metronidazole or vancomycin should be given orally – the dose of vancomycin can be as low as 250mg 6-hourly administered for 5 days. Although little difference has been demonstrated between the efficacy of these two drugs as assessed in clinical trials, many feel that for severe or relapse cases vancomycin is the better drug. In general, for most cases receiving chemotherapy, metronidazole is preferable because of its cheapness.

It may seem strange to some that diarrhoea apparently induced by one antibiotic may be improved by another. It is important to remember that pseudomembranous colitis may relapse and the true relationship of this condition to inflammatory bowel disease has not been established.

Patients who have experienced *Cl. difficile* diarrhoea caused by a particular antibiotic are apparently not at increased risk of developing diarrhoea during subsequent administration of the same drug.

OTHER CLOSTRIDIAL STRAINS

A number of clostridia, other than *Cl. difficile* are implicated in gastrointestinal disorders.

Cl. botulinum *Infection*

Botulism is a serious illness induced by ingestion of the neurotoxins of *Cl. botulinum*. Symptoms usually occur within 12 to 36 hours of taking the contaminated food which may be normal in taste and appearance. The patients are afebrile, and nausea and vomiting are the exception. Cranial nerve disorder, particularly ocular palsies, postural hypotension and dry mucus membranes may suggest the diagnosis.

Diagnosis is confirmed by demonstrating botulinus toxin in blood or body fluids. Treatment is supportive, and antitoxins may be administered. Mechanical support for ventilation is often required.

Cl. perfringens (welchii) *Infection*

Incomplete cooking of meat dishes is usually responsible for the symptoms of nausea and watery diarrhoea coming on within 8–24 hours of taking contaminated food. Fever and vomiting are uncommon. The condition is usually mild and seldom persists for more than 48 hours.

Enteritis necroticans is a necrotizing condition of the small bowel induced by *Cl. perfringens* type C producing B-toxin. The condition called 'pig-bel' is reported in outbreaks in New Guinea when vast quantities of undercooked pork are eaten. Abdominal pain, bloody diarrhoea, shock, peritonitis and death may ensue.

OTHER MICROBIAL AGENTS CAUSING DIARRHOEA

Vibrio parahaemolyticus *Infection*

This gastrointestinal upset presents with explosive watery diarrhoea coming on within 24 hours of eating crustaceans; imported oysters, eaten raw, is a common history. The organism produces a toxin and also causes small bowel inflammation.

Treatment

The treatment is supportive and symptomatic
  Isolation is not required.

Yersiniosis due to Yersinia enterocolitica

Yersinia enterocolitica is responsible for a number of syndromes of which acute gastrointestinal upset, including diarrhoea, is the commonest. This type of presentation is mostly encountered in young children in whom there is fever, and mesenteric adenotis. Adults are sometimes affected; erythema nodosum and reactive arthritis may be encountered.
  Isolation is not required.

Treatment

Treatment is supportive and symptomatic. Antibiotics, such as chloramphenicol or gentamicin are used in severe or invasive infections.

Cryptosporidiosis

Cryptosporidium is a protozoan parasite which may cause protracted diarrhoea in immunosuppressed individuals. Clindamycin and quinine have been used in treatment.

Aeromonas shigelloides can occasionally be responsible for a self-limiting gastrointestinal infection.

VIRUSES

Since the 1970s a number of viruses have been associated with outbreaks of infective diarrhoea in humans, both children and adults. The first agent to be well characterized was the Norwalk agent isolated from specimens obtained during an outbreak of diarrhoea in a school in Norwalk, Ohio. A number of similar agents responsible for diarrhoea in different geographical areas have been described. Table 5.2 summarizes the viruses responsible for diarrhoea.

Table 5.2   Viruses causing diarrhoea (after DuPont and Pickering)

Virus	Illness	Method of detection
Norwalk-like agents	epidemic diarrhoea in children and adults	immune electron microscopy
Rotavirus	children and adults affected	electron microscopy
Coronavairus		electron microscopy
Enteroviruses	viral syndromes including poliomyelitis	immune electron microscopy
Astroviruses		electron microscopy
Adenoviruses		electron microscopy
Minirotaviruses		electron microscopy
Calciviruses	winter vomiting disease	electron microscopy

Rotaviruses

Rotavirus – so called because its morphological appearance resembles a wheel with radiating spokes – although first described as a cause of infective diarrhoea in children, can also affect adults. Outbreaks in geriatric wards have been described. The incubation period for this form of diarrhoea is from 2 to 4 days. Profuse watery diarrhoea with low grade fever and vomiting are the characteristic features.

Diagnosis is most rapidly accomplished by finding rotavirus particles in stool samples by electron microscopy. Virus excretion seldom continues for longer than 8 days.

Treatment

Treatment is supportive and symptomatic.
Isolation is obligatory.

Diarrhoea is often part of a more generalized virus infection; this is particularly likely to occur with enteroviruses including poliomyelitis.

WHAT PATIENTS WITH DIARRHOEA SHOULD BE ISOLATED?

Ideally all patients with acute diarrhoea should be admitted to an isolation unit but many patients can be satisfactorily isolated at home. This permits assessment, diagnosis and management in conditions of safety with staff who are trained in the techniques of infection control. This practice indicates those patients who are a hazard in general wards – salmonella infections and bacillary dysentery are obvious examples – while those with non-infective disorders such as inflammatory bowel disease or neoplasms are referred to the appropriate departments.

If this policy, or some modification of it is not followed, the inevitable result is outbreaks of infective diarrhoea in general wards. Regrettably, this is the position which most physicians and geriatricians will encounter.

The situation is often more complex than outlined above for patients may be admitted to hospital with a major illness such as cerebrovascular accident, or a myocardial infarction, and during the course of his hospital stay diarrhoea is noted. Very often, because the diarrhoea is not very marked, it may not be recognized as infective. Should such a patient be left in the general ward, removed to a side room, or removed to an isolation unit which may be in another hospital? Each case must be assessed separately. A side room in a busy general ward is not ideal but it is often the only isolation facility which is available. In the case of a single episode of diarrhoea the diagnosis may be confirmed and appropriate action taken. If there are a number of cases of diarrhoea occurring about the same time then removal to more formal isolation becomes obligatory. Stopping admissions to the ward and treating the ward as an isolation unit with 'cohort nursing' is occasionally an acceptable compromise.

In this situation it is vital that there is co-operation between geriatricians, microbiologists, and infectious disease staff. Most hospitals now have a control-of-infection sister whose help is crucial in hospital outbreaks. It is clear that there is considerable organizational responsibility for all hospital staff to co-operate in providing an infectious disease consultation service in which problems of prevention, isolation, treatment and management can be resolved in the context of available equipment, staff and expertise.

Further Reading

DuPont, H. L. and Pickering, L. K. (1980). *Infections of the Gastrointestinal Tract*. (New York: Plenum Medical Book Company)

Rubin, R. A. and Weinstein, L. (1977). *Salmonellosis*. (New York: Stratton Intercontinental Medical Book Corporation)

Gray, J. A. and Trueman, M. (1971). Severe salmonella gastroenteritis associated with hypo-chlorhydria *Scot. Med J.* **16,** 255–8

Larson, E. H., (1979). Pseudomembranous colitis is an infection. *J. Infect,* **1,** 221–6

Lambert (ed.) (1979). *Clinics in Gastroenterology. Infections of the GI Tract*. (London: Saunders Ltd)

Brooks (ed.) (1978). *Gastrointestinal Pathophysiology, 2nd Ed.* (Oxford University Press)

Abeyesundere, R. L. (1982). A ward outbreak of *Clostridium difficile* enterocolitis. *J. Infect.,* **3,** 277–82

Editorial (1984). Unravelling the secrets of *Clostridium difficile. J. Infect.,* **8,** 97–9

6

Infections in the Abdominal Cavity in Old Age

F. D. BEGGS and A. E. KARK

There are more than 2½ million people in the United Kingdom over 75 years of age and nearly ½ million are over 85[1]. This is a four-fold increase over the same population in 1911 compared with a total population increase of one-third. Infection now ranks fourth as the cause of death in the elderly population after cancer, myocardial infarction and cerebrovascular accident. Infection is in addition a frequent end-stage event in other diseases. The elderly population is not only at greater risk of developing an infection, but has a higher mortality when infection does develop.

ATYPICAL PRESENTATION OF INFECTION IN THE ELDERLY

The characteristics and manifestations of abdominal infections in the elderly may vary dramatically from those usually encountered in younger individuals. Early diagnosis may be difficult due to abnormal presentations, particularly in those with an altered mental state (Table 6.1).

A major diagnostic trap occurs in a geriatric patient who frequently has concurrent pathological conditions of many systems, and advanced sepsis can frequently present as multiple system failure. All the abnormalities present must be diagnosed and their relative importance to the current status of a patient must be assessed. For example, the physical signs present in a patient with a perforated duodenal ulcer may be masked by steroids taken for rheumatic disease, by ischaemic heart disease resulting in a paradoxically slow pulse or the management can be complicated by chronic bronchitis. In addition, a patient who has become accustomed to the pain of severe arthritis may accept with equanimity the pain of acute calculous cholecystitis.

Table 6.1 Atypical presentations of intra-abdominal infections in old age

1. Psychiatric
   confusion
   delirium
   'acting strangely'

2. Failure to thrive
3. Anorexia and weight loss

4. Cardiorespiratory
   deteriorating congestive cardiac failure
   worsening respiratory failure
   tachycardia
   hypotension

5. Diabetic crisis

6. Urological
   frequency of micturition
   incontinence

7. Unexplained rashes
8. Cerebrovascular accident

9. Haematological
   raised white cell count
   purpura
   anaemia

DIFFICULTIES IN HISTORY-TAKING

Another diagnostic problem may be the difficulty in obtaining a clear history. Many elderly patients will deny any physical ailment requiring surgical treatment; indeed many will have memories of an era when major surgery was routinely followed by death, and will try to mislead a surgeon. Relatives or those who are close to the patient may not be available and patients are frequently sent to hospital from 'welfare home accommodation' or a nursing home accompanied by unqualified and uninformed personnel. The patient's regular practitioner will usually be able to provide valuable information, but frequently an elderly person's condition deteriorates when away from home or when the usual general practitioner is unavailable. Many a sick, elderly patient will claim never to have been ill in his life, while examination will reveal multiple abdominal operation scars.

The diagnostic difficulties in the elderly are highlighted by a study of patients with peptic ulcer perforations[2]. Many of the patients documented provided diagnostic difficulties such that they were admitted to medical wards for investigation, some of the diagnoses in fact being made in the operating theatre.

NECESSITY FOR EARLY DIAGNOSIS

There is no doubt that prompt diagnosis and management of all forms of intra-abdominal infection result in very low morbidity and mortality, even in the elderly. The critical importance of early diagnosis and treatment of intra-abdominal abscesses has been well documented by Pitcher *et al*.[3]. These authors examined the clinical course of 77 patients with intra-abdominal infection with particular attention to the effect of diagnostic and treatment delays on the incidence of complications and mortality. The overall mortality in the series was 39%, the highest mortality occurring in patients with peritonitis (64%) or intra-abdominal abscess (63%). No significant correlation was found between patient age and mortality. Mortality varied with the number of complications.

All patients who did not develop complications survived, but the mortality was 29% in patients who developed one complication, 36% in those who developed two, and 100% in those with three or more complications ($p<0.001$). The mean number of complications was 3.4 in patients who died and 0.6 in those who survived ($p<0.001$). Delay in establishing a correct diagnosis was significantly associated with an increased morbidity and mortality (see Tables 6.2 and 6.3). It can be seen that the mean interval between presentation and diagnosis was 10 days in those who survived and 25 days in those who died ($p<0.001$); the interval between presentation and definitive therapy was 15 days in survivors and 33 days in those who died ($p<0.005$).

Table 6.2   Relation between time to diagnosis, time to treatment, complications and mortality

| Complications | Patients | *Interval* (days) | | Mortality (%) |
		Presentation to diagnosis	*Presentation to treatment*	
0	30	8	13	0
1	14	12	17	29
2	11	15	27	36
3 or more	22	24	34	100
Probability (∞^2 analysis)		< 0.01	< 0.001	< 0.001

Data from Ref. 3

Table 6.3   Effect of delay in diagnosis or therapy on mortality

| | *Mean time* (days) | | *Probability* |
	Survivors	*Fatalities*	
Presentation to diagnosis	10	25	< 0.001
Presentation to definitive therapy	15	33	< 0.005
Diagnosis to definitive therapy	5	8	NS

The figures do not include cases in which diagnosis was made only at autopsy. Inclusion of these results would have made the resulting differences even more striking. (Data from Ref. 3)

These data, and those from other series, show the critical importance of early diagnosis and treatment in all patients with intra-abdominal sepsis. It should be remembered, however, that where definitive treatment requires surgery or other invasive methods as much information as possible should be available at the time of surgery to enable this to be performed effectively.

SURGERY IN THE AGED

Even in an emergency situation, age of itself has not been found to bear any correlation with operative mortality[4]. Mortality is related to the severity and nature of the surgical condition and to the intolerance of the elderly to cardiorespiratory complications. From the study of 375 patients it was concluded that:

1. a prompt and active approach to diagnosis and management must be adopted in the elderly;
2. early definitive surgery is ideal;
3. multiple staged operations are inadvisable since definitive surgery is delayed.

BACTERIOLOGY OF ABDOMINAL INFECTIONS

The common micro-organisms found in infections in the abdomen reflect the normal bacterial flora of the gastrointestinal tract (Table 6.4).

Table 6.4

Site	Bacteria
Oesophagus	*Bacteroides* spp. (except *B. fragilis*); peptostreptococci
Stomach	Sterile if empty due to gastric acidity (pH 2)
Biliary tract	Sterile in health
Duodenum Jejunum Upper ileum	Very scanty numbers increasing in the ileum to very large numbers in the colon
Colon	Non-sporing anaerobes, including *B. fragilis*, outnumbering aerobic (Gram-negative bacilli, principally *E. coli*, by 1000 to 10 000:1; faecal streptococci; *Clostridium* spp.

In the elderly, however, in whom gastric acid output is decreased, the pH rising to 4–8, the bacterial flora of the stomach will be represented by enteric Gram-negative bacilli and non-sporing anaerobes. Where gastrointestinal motility is reduced, the flora of the small bowel will resemble that of the colon. In calculous cholecystitis up to 30% of cultures of bile will contain Gram-negative coliforms and *S. faecalis*. Anaerobes are less common, being present in up to 3%.

Where there is established intra-abdominal infection, a course of antibiotic therapy is mandatory and the choice of agent(s) must be 'best-guess' based on knowledge of local microbial flora until the results of culture and sensitivity are available. In gastrointestinal surgery the choice will lie between a second- or third-generation cephalosporin, e.g. cefuroxime or ceftazidime, or an aminoglycoside together with metronidazole. In biliary surgery a Gram stain of bile at operation may influence choice. In general a second- or third-generation cephalosporin will suffice. Administration by the intravenous route is preferred in order to provide reliable tissue levels of antibiotics. The exception is metronidazole which may be given by suppository provided the patient can retain this formulation. In urologic surgery, preoperative culture of urine will dictate the appropriate agent. Where elective, clean-contaminated surgical procedures are to be performed, antibiotic prophylaxis may be indicated. In surgery, such prophylaxis means the administration of an appropriate agent(s) to patients with no evidence of established infection but in whom there is a significant risk of the development of postoperative infection.

The agent should be administered such that from the time of the surgical incision to completion of the operation, the concentration of antibiotic present in the tissues being handled is sufficient to prevent the relevant bacteria establishing infection in the wound. A bolus intravenous injection, rather than slow infusion, is preferred, timed with induction of anaesthesia, with a further dose if the procedure exceeds 2h. Continuation of prophylaxis beyond a maximum of 24h is of no value and serves only to increase the risk of drug toxicity and bacterial superinfection.

DIAGNOSTIC METHODS AVAILABLE

The method by which a clinician will reach a diagnosis of intra-abdominal sepsis will vary according to the individual clinician. In general it will proceed along conventional lines of history-taking, clinical examination and special investigations. The relative importance of each of these will vary with the individual enquirer.

History

As previously stated, taking a history in the elderly may be fraught with difficulties such as deafness, dementia and confusion. If a clear, reliable history were available, there would be few diagnostic difficulties. Consequently history-taking should not be confined to one individual; the patient and the relatives should be questioned and occasionally more than one clinician should extract the history. Clues such as a 'chill' (fever) or dark urine (jaundice or dehydration) should be sought carefully, and intelligent use made of as many leading questions as possible.

Examination

Physical findings may differ from those expected. Slight localized tenderness may be the only evidence of serious intra-abdominal pathology. There may be no evidence of shock, rigidity, distension or guarding. The patient may spike a low-grade pyrexia or may be apyrexial. A high index of suspicion and an awareness of the possibility of intra-abdominal sepsis are frequently the only features that aid a diagnosis. It should be remembered that the elderly population has already been naturally selected by epidemics and two World Wars, and must not necessarily be regarded as frail. They may be unusually stoical.

Whatever the mental state of the patient, much can be learned from observing the patient closely whilst taking an unhurried history. Valuable diagnostic clues, such as the nature of vomitus, can easily be missed if an incontinent patient is cleaned by the nursing staff before examination. The characteristics of respiration and the willingness of the patient to move should also be noted. A patient with severe intra-abdominal pathology rarely moves or breathes freely. An unwillingness to cough may particularly be related to peritonitis. When free gas is present in the peritoneal cavity, the abdomen may become distended and tympanitic and liver dullness may be lost. The general state of the patient will frequently raise the possibility of intra-abdominal pathology. The examination is not complete without a rectal examination, which will not only reveal pelvic tenderness due to sepsis but may yield information about other conditions such as faecal impaction.

Laboratory Investigations

Blood samples should be obtained for routine laboratory investigation, including haemoglobin estimation, white cell count and the measurement of urea, amylase and electrolytes. The results of these investigations will not establish the specific diagnosis of abdominal sepsis but may give information about other conditions which will provide an alternative diagnosis, or may at least confirm the presence of organic pathology. The serum amylase must be interpreted with caution unless it is sufficiently elevated to be diagnostic of pancreatitis.

Blood cultures, preferably three sets, should be performed on the merest suspicion of sepsis. Ideally they should be taken from separate sites during a pyrexia. Identification and evaluation of any organism grown may indicate a starting point for investigations.

General Radiological Examination

Many difficulties exist in the radiological evaluation of the elderly patient.

Poor co-operation, immobility and hypotension may make the radiological examination difficult to perform, particularly during hours when fewer personnel are available. In these circumstances the clinician should make every effort to accompany the patient to the radiology department and to ensure that the films are the best that can be obtained and hence provide as much information as possible. Plain chest and abdominal radiographs may be of direct diagnostic value (Table 6.5) in up to 50% of patients[5].

Table 6.5 Signs present on plain chest and abdominal films

1. Obvious:	Free gas – perforation
	Gallstones
	Renal or ureteric calculi
	Appendicular faecolith
2. Subtle:	Sympathetic pleural effusions, e.g. pancreatitis
	Elevation/fixation of diaphragm, e.g. subphrenic abscess
	Soft tissue mass, e.g. bladder, ovarian cyst
	Displacement of viscera
	Localized ileus, e.g. appendicitis
	Loss of definition of retroperitoneal structures, e.g. psoas abscess

Value of Diagnostic Paracentesis

This is a valuable and often essential procedure to help diagnose intra-peritoneal infections, especially when there are no localized collections. The procedure has the following advantages:

1. The test can be performed immediately at the bedside.
2. The procedure disturbs the patient far less than the manipulations required to obtain satisfactory radiographs.
3. Paracentesis can be extremely useful in hospitals with limited radiographic facilities, particularly during non-peak hours.
4. The procedure is associated with a yield of positive information that is at least comparable to that provided by radiological techniques.
5. Safety.

A negative paracentesis, however, has no significance. The results of paracentesis are more likely to be positive when the peritoneal cavity contains more than 500 ml of fluid. The safety of paracentesis has been questioned, particularly in patients with intestinal obstruction. This complaint has been investigated experimentally and reviewed clinically. The conclusion is that leakage from accidental bowel perforation is a very small hazard indeed. As a precautionary measure, however, paracentesis should not be performed in the presence of a distended bowel.

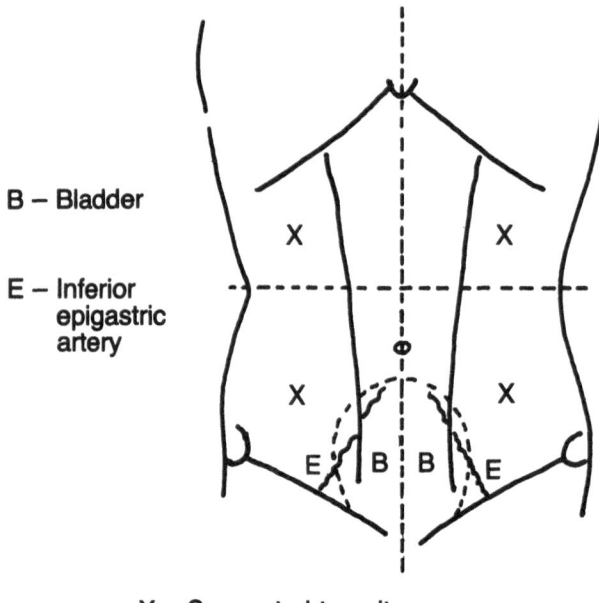

B – Bladder

E – Inferior
epigastric
artery

X – Suggested tap sites

Figure 6.1 Sites of puncture in the standard four-quadrant tap

Technique

The standard technique used in paracentesis is a four-quadrant tap (Figure 6.1). A 2 ml or 5 ml disposable syringe and a 21 gauge needle are used. Local anaesthesia is not necessary. The procedure is performed with clean hands after the skin has been washed with an alcohol and chlorhexidine preparation.

The needle is advanced rapidly through the skin in order to minimize discomfort. Thereafter the needle is slowly advanced while applying suction with the syringe. The patient will experience discomfort as the parietal peritoneum is punctured, the tip of the needle is moved about inside the peritoneal cavity and a sample of fluid is aspirated. Once a positive result is obtained, no other site need be tapped. If the tap is negative, the test is repeated in another quadrant until positive, or until all quadrants have been tapped.

Results

In the absence of intra-abdominal sepsis or other pathology, less than 0.5 ml of clear peritoneal fluid may be obtained. When a larger quantity of fluid is obtained, an underlying cause nearly always exists. The number of tests performed on the aspirate will depend on the type and amount of the fluid and of the experience of the observer[6].

1. *Purulent or seropurulent material:* a smear should be Gram stained and examined under a microscope. Pus cells will confirm an inflammatory reaction. The presence of Gram-negative rods will indicate a gastrointestinal perforation.
2. *Fresh blood:* this will require no more tests.
3. *Thin, dark blood:* a smear for organisms and an amylase estimation should be performed. In cases of devitalized gut there is a characteristic odour to the fluid.
4. *Serous fluid:* this may result from extravasation of urine, ruptured cysts, acute pancreatitis etc.
5. *Bile:* this is usually recognized by its colour and can be confirmed by biochemical tests.
6. *Faeces:* this is somewhat worrying to the observer, implying that he has perforated the bowel. If the tap has been correctly performed, it is most likely to have come from free faeces in the peritoneal cavity and the degree of illness of the patient will be corroborative evidence.
7. *Chylous peritoneal fluid:* this is usually recognizable, but can be confirmed by a fat stain.

Paracentesis is a simple and safe procedure. It is most useful when the results are positive. When negative, however, paracentesis proves nothing. Some authors favour the more complicated technique of peritoneal lavage using a peritoneal dialysis cannula. Although the diagnostic yield is generally higher, so is the complication rate. In such situations the procedure of choice may be laparoscopy or laparotomy.

LOCALIZATION OF INTRA-ABDOMINAL ABSCESS

Despite the utilization of the simple diagnostic methods described above, some patients will remain unwell for no obvious cause. In these patients an intra-abdominal abscess must be suspected, walled off from the rest of the peritoneal cavity. These abscesses may be solitary or multiloculated, within the peritoneal cavity itself or in the adjacent retroperitoneum.

Intra-abdominal abscesses arise in four ways:

1. Those arising during resolution and healing of generalized peritonitis.
2. Those that result from perforation of the gastrointestinal and biliary tract, successfully walled off in the acute stage by peritoneal defence mechanisms.
3. Those which develop within the solid viscera after haematogenous or lymphatic dissemination of infection from a septic focus elsewhere in the body.

4. Retroperitoneal abscesses which arise as a consequence of primary infection or inflammation of the retroperitoneal viscera followed by secondary bacterial contamination.

There are a number of potential locations for intra-abdominal abscess. (see Table 6.6).

Table 6.6 Distribution and frequency of intra-abdominal abscesses

Subphrenic	30%
Pelvic	25%
Paracolic	12%
Periappendicular	12%
Intermesenteric	5%
Lesser sac	5%
Hepatic	1%

^{67}Ga Citrate Scan

A variety of new imaging techniques is available to aid the clinician. Originally used as a tumour scanning agent, gallium-67 was later found to localize inflammatory foci. Its accuracy rate is about 80% but it has a number of drawbacks:

1. following intravenous injection the majority of ^{67}Ga citrate is excreted via the intestines and, despite cleansing bowel enemas, intestinal accumulations may result in a false-positive;
2. 48–72 hours delay between injection and scanning may be necessary to diminish background radiation and this delay may be unacceptable;
3. the technique does not distinguish between inflammation and pus.

The value of the test is that it may indicate a starting point for further investigation by means of ultrasound and computerized tomography. Its main advantage is that the whole body image may reveal septic foci outside the abdominal cavity.

^{111}In-labelled Leukocytes

Autologous leukocytes labelled with indium-111 are accurate in 92% of cases of intra-abdominal abscess. Studies can be more rapid than with gallium-67, being completed within 24h. In addition, a false-positive is less likely as the leukocytes are not excreted via the gut. Inflammatory bowel disease can, in theory, be a problem, but in practice this is not so. Indium-labelled leukocytes do not accumulate in a normally healing wound and an abscess deep to an infected wound can usually be identified using lateral views. The principal disadvantage of the technique is that leukocytes accumulate in the spleen and the presence of splenunculi may be wrongly diagnosed as being an abscess. Its principal use is probably now as a starting point for more definitive investigation.

Ultrasound

Grey-scale ultrasonography has been used with considerable success in the detection of intra-abdominal abscesses. With suitable care and experience in the interpretation of the image obtained it is possible to differentiate the appearance of an abscess, which is typically rounded, with slightly irregular walls, and contains weakly echogenic debris, from other intra-abdominal fluid collections.

Real-time ultrasonography can help to distinguish fluid-filled loops of bowel by revealing peristaltically induced movement of echogenic particles within the lumen. The technique is rapid and non-invasive, involves no ionizing radiation and is relatively inexpensive and widely available. It is, however, completely dependent on operator skill and interpretation. A further advantage is that ultrasound may be used to guide needle aspiration of a suspected abscess cavity thus providing immediate confirmation of the diagnosis (Table 6.7), particularly in those cases where the appearances are doubtful or the patients are critically ill. However there are several limitations to its use:

1. Scattering of the sound beam occurs in obese patients, often giving rise to unsatisfactory scans.
2. Intestinal gas reflects the sound beam, thus obscuring the view of deeper structures. It may, for example, be impossible to obtain a satisfactory scan in a patient with a paralytic ileus and the presence of gas in the stomach and transverse colon may obscure the view in the left upper quadrant.
3. Open wounds, colostomies, drains or dressings may also limit the completeness of the examination.

Despite these drawbacks, the accuracy of grey scale ultrasound in detecting intra-abdominal abscesses has been reported to be from 90% to 96% in several different series.

CT Scanning

The use of computerized tomography has now been well evaluated in the diagnosis of intra-abdominal abscess, with an accuracy rate of over 95%

(Table 6.7). An abscess appears on the CT scan as a low-density mass. Abnormal collection of gas within the lesion is found in up to 50% of cases and rim enhancement occurs in 30–40%. It is necessary to administer contrast medium orally prior to the examination in order to distinguish fluid-filled loops of bowel from abscesses. However the appearances are not absolutely specific for abscesses and may mimic haematomas, seromas or even a diffuse inflammatory reaction. Therefore it is necessary to correlate CT appearances closely with the clinical findings.

CT scans appear to have some unique advantages in the management of intra-abdominal abscess:

1. Those patients who, although demonstrating no localizing signs, are suspected of harbouring septic foci intra-abdominally.
2. CT is superior to ultrasound in patients suspected of having a pelvic abscess. In this situation pelvic ultrasound is difficult due to interference from pelvic bones.
3. CT is superior in multiple and deep-seated abdominal lesions, especially those lying in close proximity to the gastrointestinal tract.

Where CT scanning is employed to look for an abscess, it is the definitive investigation in up to 70% of cases.

Table 6.7 Comparative indications for ultrasound or CT scanning for abscess location

Ultrasound	CT Scanning
Localized collection suspected clinically	Suspected pelvic abscess
Adjunct to percutaneous drainage	Suspected multiple abscesses Inter-loop abscesses

Derived from Sani *et al.* (1983)
Am. J. Surg., **145**(1), 136–42

THE DIAGNOSTIC ROLE OF SURGERY

Unfortunately, in many institutions the full range of investigative methods is not available. All hospitals, however, have access to a surgeon and in many cases a diagnostic laparoscopy or laparotomy will be indicated.

Laparoscopy

This is an appropriate course of action for confirmation of an uncertain diagnosis and collection of intra-abdominal bacteriological specimens. It is contraindicated in the presence of generalized peritonitis or bowel distension, both of which make laparotomy a safer and more useful alternative.

The technique is less likely to be of value in the elderly in whom a laparotomy is more appropriate.

Laparotomy

This is a safe procedure requiring few specialized instruments. It is assumed that full investigation of an elderly patient will have resulted in no diagnosis being made. Laparotomy can be swiftly performed in almost all patients through a mid-line incision. It is preferable, however, only to reach this stage when all reasonable alternatives have been tried and when it is performed for the potential benefit of the patient and not for the clinician's interest.

The mortality and morbidity of a negative laparotomy is extremely low. It allows all aspects of the abdomen to be both inspected and palpated for pathology. Its advantage is speed, and the possibility for definitive surgery or drainage to be performed at the same time. Most of the morbidity and mortality associated with a laparotomy will be due to the definitive procedure performed and its complications rather than to the incision itself. Nevertheless the procedure should not be lightly undertaken; a negative laparotomy will not help the patient and it should not be performed until all reasonable preoperative investigations have been completed.

SALIENT FEATURES AND DIAGNOSTIC DIFFICULTIES OF SOME CONDITIONS

Bowel

Perforated Peptic Ulcer

Although perforation in the elderly will occasionally present with the typical history of sudden onset of severe pain and marked abdominal rigidity on palpation, with the diagnosis being confirmed by the presence of gas under the diaphragm, in others, signs and symptoms are non-specific and diagnostic clues are absent or muted.

Factors contributing to increased mortality in elderly patients with perforated peptic ulcers include concurrent medical disease, shock and long-standing perforation (Figures 6.2a and 6.2b). Patients with mental disorders are at particularly high risk of misdiagnosis because they are usually less able to provide a coherent history and their psychiatric condition may make physical examination difficult. Surgical intervention is the only sure method of treatment, the mortality increasing with both advancing age and diagnostic delay.

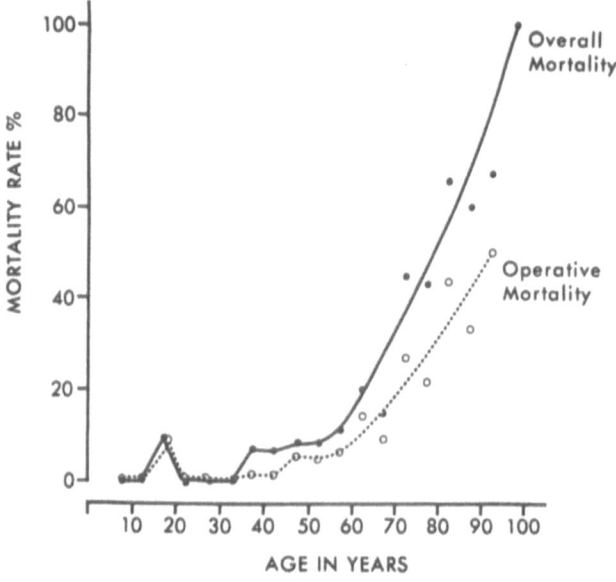

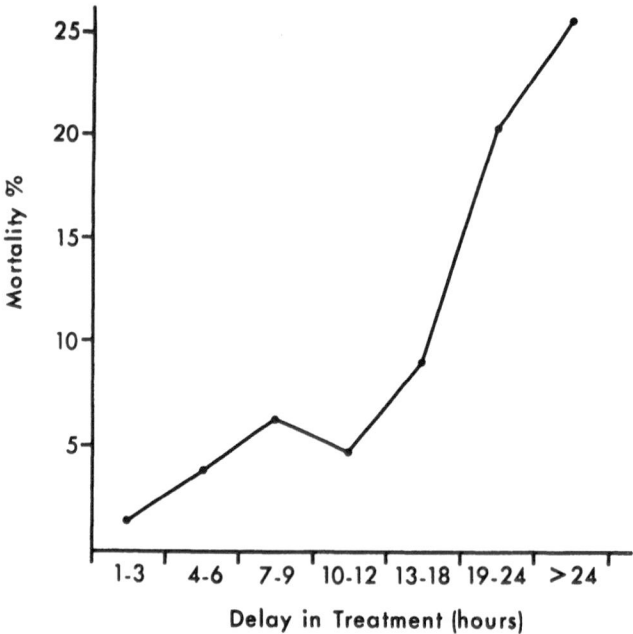

Figure 6.2 (A) Relationship between mortality resulting from perforated peptic ulcer and age. (B) Relationship between mortality resulting from perforated peptic ulcer and the delay in surgical treatment. (Adapted from Cohen, M. M. (1971) *Can. Med. Assoc. J.,* **105,** 263)

Early diagnosis is only possible if the clinician is aware of the possibility of perforation in non-specific presentation. Erect chest or lateral decubitus radiographs may demonstrate the presence of free gas, or more sophisticated techniques may be necessary to demonstrate a pneumoperitoneum. Aerated drinks or effervescent tablets may be used, but it is probably more reliable to pass a nasogastric tube. The quantity of aspirate can be very informative: if a large amount is aspirated, a perforated peptic ulcer is unlikely. If no fluid is obtained a perforated ulcer is likely. If the diagnosis is still in doubt, air can be injected down the nasogastric tube and an erect chest film repeated. Finally, gastrografin can be swallowed by the patient, or passed down the nasogastric tube, and a perforation visualized either directly, on screening, or indirectly by the late appearance of a nephrogram.

Abdominal paracentesis is particularly useful when perforation is suspected, the technique being quick, safe and producing a high diagnostic yield. Very occasionally, a small leak will become walled off by omentum and the patient will present with clinical signs of a chest infection. Chest radiograph will reveal basal collapse and a small effusion. Subsequent investigation by ultrasonography will reveal a subphrenic collection and this can either be drained surgically or by means of a catheter placed under radiographic control.

Where a frank perforation is present, surgery is mandatory, however high the operative risk. Nevertheless, a few hours can be spent correcting fluid balance and generally making the patient as fit for surgery as possible. Frequent nasogastric aspiration and intravenous antibiotics are essential measures to prepare the patient for surgery. Where an acute ulcer only is found at laparotomy this should be closed by direct suture reinforced by omentum and peritoneal lavage carried out by means of saline and suction. Where the ulcer is chronic, and the patient's general condition permits, peritoneal soiling is minimal, and where both operator and anaesthetist are sufficiently experienced, consideration can be given to performing definitive surgery for the underlying lesion. It is preferable that only one operation is performed in the elderly, if present and future problems can be corrected without increasing mortality and morbidity.

Inflammatory Bowel Disease

Both Crohn's disease and ulcerative colitis are generally conditions associated with younger patients. Consequently, the relatively small number of elderly patients who develop inflammatory bowel disease later in life are at a greater risk of missed diagnosis. This diagnostic difficulty will result in delay of specific treatment and this may help explain the high mortality rates reported in these patients[7].

The diagnosis of inflammatory bowel disease can be established by clinical behaviour, sigmoidoscopic appearance and barium enema or small bowel enema. In view of the potential diagnostic difficulties, however, the opportunity should be taken, on proctoscopy, to perform a rectal biopsy. This may result in a diagnosis being made before it is clinically apparent. There are several differences in the behaviour of inflammatory bowel disease in the elderly. In the older age group, unlike the young, proctitis will be due to Crohn's disease in approximately half the cases. A variable number of these will require surgery to control their symptoms. The uncommon complications of inflammatory bowel disease, toxic dilatation, free perforation and massive haemorrhage are very much more common in the elderly in whom such complications have a very high mortality. Early surgical treatment has been advocated in the elderly; certainly early surgery performed electively before the development of septic complications can result in improved survival[8].

Appendicitis

The incidence of appendicitis in the elderly has risen steadily as a result of increasing longevity. Elderly women are more likely than the young to have appendicitis than a pain of gynaecological origin. The mortality of older patients with appendicitis is seven times that of the younger patients[9]. This high mortality is chiefly a result of delay in definitive treatment together with the lowered physiological reserves of the elderly. Cardiac disease and pulmonary emboli are the main direct causes of death.

Several studies have shown that the inflamed appendix is more often perforated in old than in young patients, indeed more than 30–40% have a perforated appendix at the time of surgery. Impaired blood supply and structural weakness of the appendix are likely to produce earlier perforation in the elderly. Atherosclerosis of the appendicular artery probably results in rapid gangrene of an inflamed, obstructed appendix.

Despite a strongly suggestive history with supporting physical signs, most series show that the appendix is normal in 25–30% of patients who have surgery and this rises to 40–50% in the elderly. A need therefore exists to improve the accuracy of the clinical diagnosis. Unfortunately no reliable special investigations exist to solve the problem, and the diagnosis of acute appendicitis in the elderly is based primarily on history and physical findings. Arnbjornsson[10] compared the relative frequency of the physical signs in elderly patients with appendicitis with the signs in young adults. The only consistent significant finding was pain and tenderness in the right iliac fossa on deep palpation. This was present in most cases. The classic history of central pain moving to the right iliac fossa was present in only 41% and rebound tenderness in the right iliac fossa was present in a significantly lower percentage of elderly patients. The classic signs of pain, anorexia and nausea were present in most of the older patients but were less pronounced than in the younger patients. Pain in the lower right quadrant was the most frequent

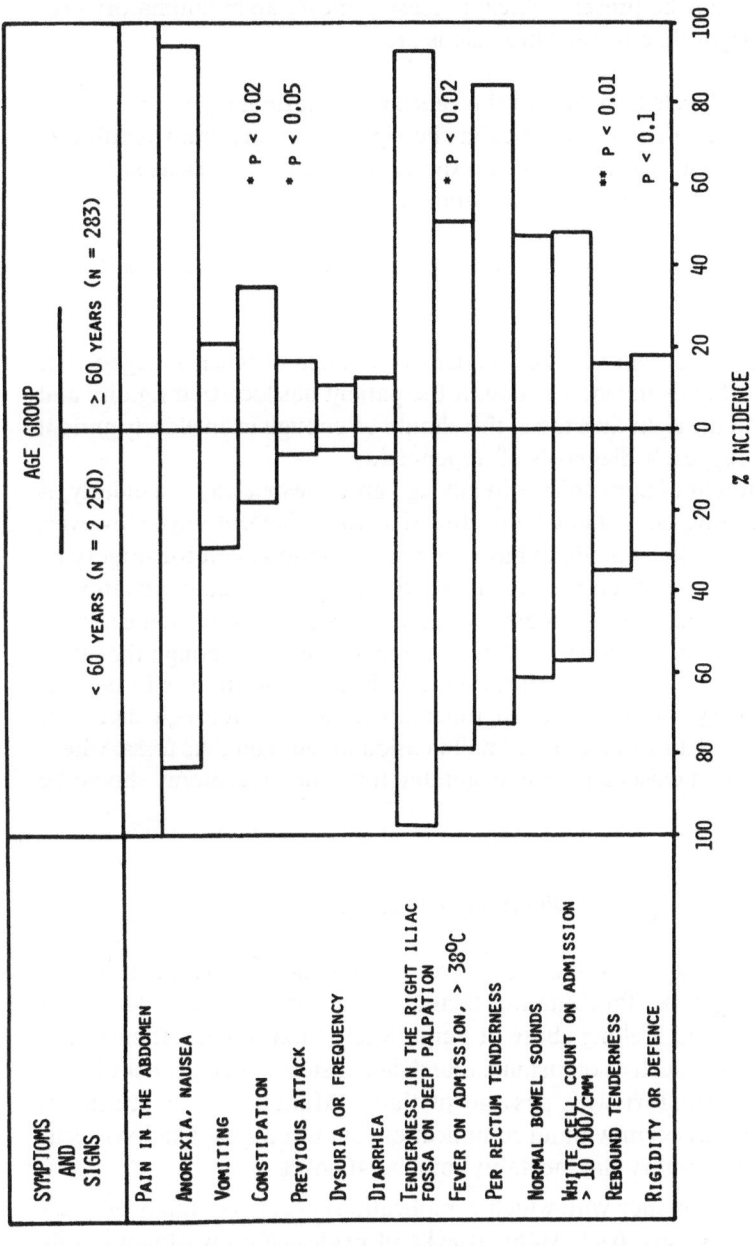

Figure 6.3 The symptoms and signs of 283 patients, 60 years of age and older, as compared with younger adults, 15–60 years of age. Patients underwent surgery at the Department of Surgery, University of Lund, Lund, Sweden, from 1969 to 1982. A statistically significant difference between these two groups was found with regard to the distribution of signs and symptoms (chi-square test, $p < 0.001$). From Arnbjornsson, E. (1984), *Geriat. Med. Today*, **3**, 72–9

complaint but was often mild and caused little concern (Figure 6.3).

The plain abdominal radiograph can occasionally be helpful; a number of appearances may be present which, at least, indicate an inflammatory process in the right iliac fossa. These signs are:

1. air-fluid levels localized to the caecum and terminal ileum;
2. increased soft tissue density in the right lower quadrant tending to obscure the sacroiliac joint on the right or the right psoas shadow;
3. appendicoliths or a gas-filled appendix;
4. deformity of the caecum;
5. free gas in the peritoneum, outside the bowel or in the retroperitoneal space

These radiological signs may occasionally be enough to clinch a diagnosis of appendicitis, but even when absent, if the patient has localized rigidity and tenderness in the right iliac fossa, this should be enough in an elderly patient to strongly suggest a diagnosis of appendicitis.

The treatment of appendicitis in any age group, especially the elderly, is appendicectomy, no patient being too sick for a laparotomy. However, every effort should be made to have the patient optimally fit for surgery by careful correction of fluid and electrolyte balance and the administration of suitable antibiotics, notably metronidazole and a broad-spectrum cephalosporin, e.g. cefuroxine or ceftazidime, or aminoglycoside, though the latter should be used with caution in the elderly if administration is to be prolonged. Surgery should not be significantly delayed. Although there are obvious surgical advantages to a small incision in the right iliac fossa, where diagnostic doubt exists an incision suitable for a full laparotomy should be performed.

Diverticular Disease

Some degree of diverticular disease is common in the elderly, the incidence possibly being 50%. Precipitating factors are a low-fibre diet, decreased body mobility and lifelong abuse of purgatives[11]. Many older patients have minor symptoms such as occasional diarrhoea, distension and colicky lower abdominal discomfort with passage of flatus. Multiple minor attacks of diverticulitis may occur without complication, but when complications occur which require surgery the mortality may be 40–60%.

The actual frequency with which complications occur is virtually impossible to assess (Figure 6.4). Many attacks of even acute diverticulitis will subside spontaneously. The attack resembles an attack of left-sided appendicitis and the point at which the complications become life-threatening can be difficult to define. For this reason all attacks should be regarded as potentially serious; the patient should be hospitalized and treated by starvation, possibly nasogastric intubation, intravenous fluids, analgesics and antibiotics including metronidazole. If the condition settles, the immediate future management should not involve surgery. In such a patient, further diagnostic information must be sought by means of barium enema or colonoscopy to ensure that the true diagnosis is not colonic carcinoma. If the symptoms fail to subside, emergency surgery is indicated, and this will usually involve resection of the affected segment of bowel, peritoneal lavage and the formation of a temporary colostomy. The precise procedure will depend on the state of the patient and the skill of the surgeon.

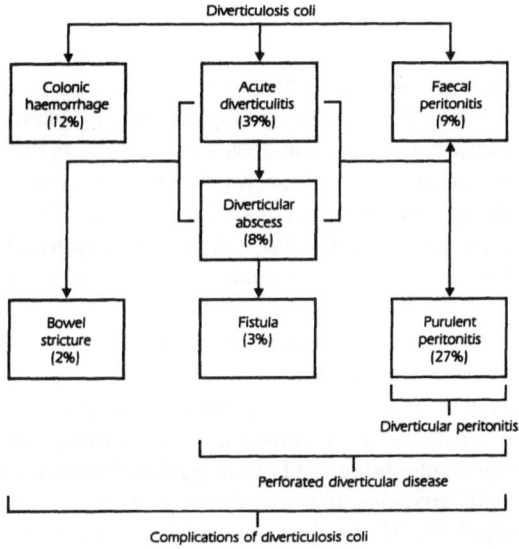

Figure 6.4 Incidence of complications of diverticular disease in 190 consecutive admissions to Crawley and Redhill hospitals (population 330 000) over a 10-year period, 1971 to 1980. (From: Smallwood, J. A. (1982) *Hospital Update,* 1554-61)

Ischiorectal Abscess

Where a diagnosis of pyrexia of undetermined origin exists in an elderly patient the possibility of an ischiorectal abscess should be actively excluded. Deep-seated abscess can be easily overlooked; pain in this area being attributed to early decubitus ulcers. A careful and unhurried rectal examination must be performed and the ischiorectal fossae carefully palpated for evidence of tenderness. If left, such abscesses can attain huge dimensions and produce the complications of fistulous tracts to the rectum or urethra. Early surgery is obviously curative and preventive.

Gall bladder

The incidence of gallstones increases from 27% between the ages of 60 and 70, to 40% over the age of 70[12]. Thus, acute cholecystitis is a common surgical emergency in the elderly, requiring admission. More seriously, gallstone disease may present, especially in the elderly, as septicaemic shock from acute suppurative ascending cholangitis. Such patients will characteristically present with abdominal pain, fever, jaundice, mental confusion and shock. They are usually elderly and the mortality may be as high as 60%[13]. Rapid diagnosis and prompt management are of prime importance. Several diagnostic procedures including oral cholecystogram, cholescintigraphy, intravenous cholangiography, ultrasonography and infusion tomography need to be considered. Down et al.[14] recently reported a sensitivity of 75% and a specificity of 82% for oral cholecystography. The procedure requires adequate liver function and a patent cystic duct for demonstration of gall bladder stones. Acutely ill patients will not be able to tolerate oral intake and repeat examination is required in 25%, thus extending the time required for diagnosis. Intravenous cholangiography has been used to diagnose acute cholecystitis for many years, but carries a 10–20% morbidity and a 0.02% mortality with a sensitivity of only 65%[15]. A further additional disadvantage is that 24h may be necessary for adequate visualization of the biliary tree.

Hepatobiliary scintigraphy has proved to be a rapid, non-invasive and sensitive method of diagnosing acute cholecystitis. A predictive value as high as 96.6% has been reported from many centres even in patients with acalculous cholecystitis. A normal hepatobiliary scan in the elderly can be of immense value in preventing an unnecessary operation. The above three methods all give indirect evidence of cholecystitis. Contrast tomography of the gall bladder wall provides direct evidence of acute cholecystitis. It is a rapid procedure of about 30min duration and has a morbidity approximating that of the IVU (1/40 000). The examination is not hindered by a raised serum bilirubin. The detection of gallstones on ultrasound is well established. However the mere presence of gallstones does not indicate cholecystitis even in the presence of right upper quadrant pain. Ultrasonography will, however, demonstrate the presence of oedema of the gall bladder wall in 52% of cases of acute cholecystitis. It is likely that a combination of ultrasonography with cholescintigraphy will result in a safe and accurate diagnosis.

Early surgical intervention is the treatment of choice in acute cholecystitis. This results in a considerably shorter total hospital stay without an increase in morbidity and mortality compared with conservative management. Of patients treated conservatively 13.8% will need emergency surgery and 11.8% will not return for definitive surgery after an acute attack has settled. Early operation avoids the hazards of diagnostic error and recurrence during the waiting period. Unsuspected operative findings supporting a policy of early surgery are partial gangrene of the gall bladder, empyema, abscess walled off by omentum and frank perforation. Antibiotics, e.g. second- or third-generation cephalosporin with possibly ampicillin, should be commenced prior to surgery, which in most cases should be cholecystectomy. Controversy exists as to whether this is more difficult than the elective operation. Cholecystostomy is an alternative to be recommended where technical difficulty or a very frail patient exists. Early cholecystectomy is to be avoided in those with pancreatitis due to gallstones until the serum amylase has returned to normal. The mortality rate varies in the literature from 0 to 20% with an age-associated high incidence. The usual cause of death is operative delay, sepsis, pulmonary or cardiac problems. Ways of reducing morbidity and mortality can be deduced from this.

Urological Infections

Urinary tract infections, particularly cystitis, are extremely common diseases of aged individuals. The incidence in ambulatory women over 70 is estimated at 30% and this rises to 100% in individuals catheterized over lengthy periods and in long-stay institutions. With advancing age there is a high incidence of anatomical and physiological abnormalities including bladder outflow obstruction due to enlarged prostate or urethral stricture, bladder dysfunction, tumours and renal tract calculi. All these will result in abnormalities of urinary flow and an increased incidence of urinary tract infection. However the mere presence of organisms in a midstream (non-catheter) specimen of urine of an elderly patient is so common that it should not automatically be assumed to be the cause of a septicaemia or of abdominal pain in the elderly; frank septicaemia will only occur as a result of trauma or instrumentation of the urinary tract. Of particular importance, however, is the long-established relationship between renal calculi and *Proteus* spp. Unfortunately the elderly have poor reserves against Gram-negative urinary infections and obstruction due to a calculus will more often result in pyonephrosis.

Perinephric abscess may result from extension of a cortical, appendicular or diverticular abscess, from haematogenous spread, via periureteral lymphatics or from undue delay in draining a pyonephrosis. As in all abdominal infections in the elderly, the classic symptoms and signs of swinging pyrexia, rigidity, tenderness and fullness in the loin may not be evident in the elderly. The diagnosis will only be made by a combination of clinical awareness and the utilization of special tests, notably ultrasonography of the renal area. Treatment is by drainage, with antibiotic therapy. Drainage has traditionally been surgical, but some centres now advocate repeated aspirations under ultrasound control. After the acute situation has settled, the problem frequently remains, however, in defining the primary pathology which resulted in the abscess and this may require sophisticated radiological combined examinations.

CONCLUSIONS

Over the past 5 years major improvements in imaging techniques have taken place and this has led to percutaneous techniques for drainage of abscesses. The new developments are particularly valuable for multiple abscesses which can often be drained percutaneously. A recent study by Halasz and van Sonnenberg[16] concluded that ultrasonography or computerized tomography-guided percutaneous drainage was highly satisfactory for the definitive treatment of single, accessible collections. Complex, multilocular and phlegmonous lesions were also suitable for percutaneous drainage as a temporary measure. Inaccessible, ill-defined abscesses or those containing a large amount of necrotic material, or those that have not responded to percutaneous drainage, require formal surgical exploration with the maximum amount of preoperative information. With collaboration between physician, surgeon, radiologists and microbiologists, the incidence of missed intra-abdominal infections should be low, and the outlook should be improved.

References

1. Great Britain: Office of Population Consensus and Surveys (1975) (London: HMSO)
2. Coleman, J. A. and Denham, M. J. (1980). Perforation of peptic ulceration in the elderly. *Age Ageing*, **9**, 257
3. Pitcher, W. D. and Musher, D. M. (1982). Clinical importance of early diagnosis and treatment of intra abdominal infection. *Arch. Surg.*, **117**, 328–33
4. Blake, R. and Lynn, J. (1976). Emergency abdominal surgery in the aged. *Br. J. Surg.*, **63**, 956–60
5. Thakur, M. L., Coleman, R. E. and Welch, M. J. (1977). Indium 111 labelled leukocytes for the localisation of abscesses. *J. Lab. Clin. Med.*, **89**, 217–28
6. Giacobine, J. W. and Siler, V. E. (1960). Evaluation of diagnostic abdominal paracentesis with experimental and clinical studies. *Surg. Gynecol. Obstet.*, **110**, 676–86
7. Diethelm, A. G., Nickel, W. F. and Wantz, G. E. (1968). Ulcerative colitis in the elderly patient. *Surg. Gynecol. Obstet.*, **126**, 1223–9
8. Goligher, J. C., Hoffman, D. C. and de Dombal, F. T. (1970). Surgical treatment of severe attacks of ulcerative colitis with special reference to the advantages of early operations. *Br. Med. J.*, **4**, 703–6
9. Peltokallio, P. and Jauhianen, K. (1970). Acute appendicitis in the aged patient. *Arch. Surg.*, **100**, 140
10. Arnbjornsson, E. (1984). Recognising appendicitis in the elderly. *Geriat. Med. Today*, **3**, 72–9
11. Vowles, K. J. D. (1979). *Surgical Problems in the Aged*. pp. 116–20. (Bristol: John Wright & Sons Ltd)
12. Glen, F. and Dillon, L. D. (1978). Developing trends in acute cholecystitis in the elderly. *Arch. Surg.*, **113**, 1149–52
13. Dow, R. W. and Lindenauer, S. M. (1969). Acute obstructive suppurative cholangitis. **169**, 272–6
14. Down, R. H., Arnold, J., Goldin, A., Watts, J. McK. and Bennes, G. (1979). Comparison of accuracy of ^{99m}Tc-pyridoxylidine glutamate scanning with oral cholecystography and ultrasonography in diagnosis of acute cholecystitis. *Lancet*, **2**, 1094–7
15. Cheung, L. Y. and Chang, F. C. (1978). Intravenous cholangiography in the diagnosis of acute cholecystitis. *Arch. Surg.*, **113**, 568–70
16. Halasz, N. A. and van Sonnenberg, E. (1983). Drainage of intra-abdominal abscess. *Am. J. Surg.*, **146**, 112–15

7

Tuberculosis in the Elderly

J. E. KASIK

INTRODUCTION

Tuberculosis is a classic example of a disease that can have a long latent period between infection and clinically evident disease. After the initial infection, the disease can become quiescent and remain dormant for a variable period of time, sometimes forever. Because of this behaviour, most individuals who have become infected can be at risk for clinical disease at any time, particularly if debilitated or immunosuppressed[1].

The mode of transmission of tuberculosis is almost always by inhalation of an aerosol containing viable members of the species, *Mycobacterium tuberculosis*. The aerosol is generated by a person who has active pulmonary tuberculosis. Usually they have one or more cavitary lesions which produce secretions containing the micro-organism; and since these secretions irritate the bronchi, it induces a chronic cough which generates the infected aerosol. This aerosol is in the form of droplets which gradually lose water and become smaller until they reach 0.5–10 μm in diameter, a size which, if inhaled, can reach the alveolus. Droplets which are larger are filtered or impacted in the upper airway or bronchi and are brought up and eliminated from the body. Particles smaller than 0.5 μm do not settle out in the alveoli or respiratory bronchi and are re-exhaled[2].

When infected droplets reach the respiratory units and lodge, the mycobacteria multiply and produce a localized infection attracting macrophages and other phagocytic cells resulting in a pulmonary infiltrate[3, 4]. If the individual has been previously exposed to mycobacteria and has established immunity, the activated cells eliminate the infection.

If the individual has never been previously exposed to appropriate mycobacteria and lacks immunity, the bacteria usually continue to multiply. The infection produces an increasing number of viable organisms since the host response is different from the immunized individual. Caseation and cavitation or granuloma formation are absent in the non-immune patient, and the mononuclear cells attracted to the area may ingest the organisms but fail to kill them. Some of the organisms are carried to the regional lymph nodes where satellite foci develop. In turn, mycobacteria escape from these nodes and enter the venous circulation via the thoracic duct. As a result, these organisms are spread throughout the body and lodge in a variety of potential target organs such as the brain, spleen, bone, kidney, and other areas of the lung[2,3,5].

While this is transpiring in the normal individual, thymus-dependent, cell-mediated immunity develops and the infection is controlled. Along with the development of this immunity, monocytic cells become more numerous and kill ingested mycobacteria. The typical microscopic pathology of tuberculosis appears with epitheloid giant cells, and caseation[4].

In most instances, the infected individual who has this primary infection and develops an appropriate immune response recovers uneventfully and often without outward manifestations of illness. A few may develop a tuberculous pleural effusion or meningitis, since these forms of tuberculosis are more common following primary infection. Most of the rest do well[2,6].

There are two remnants of this usually uneventful chain of events which are clinically important. The patient develops a cell-mediated immunity and will react to the purified protein derivative (PPD) of *M. tuberculosis,* and as a remnant of the primary infection, scattered foci of live *M. tuberculosis* remain throughout the body, often for life. Thus, the person with a positive reaction to PPD has viable mycobacteria foci scattered through various organs of the body which remain there for decades; and these organisms can multiply at any time.

In most instances, these foci remain inactive; but on occasion they begin to multiply, producing disease, usually in the lung. Since immunity has been established, the typical pathology of tuberculosis appears with a fibrous, caseous, cavitary lesion. Cough and mycobacteria in the sputa ensue and the individual becomes infectious[2,5].

If these principles are recognized and understood, the events surrounding the problem involved in clinical tuberculosis in the elderly are predictable and logical:

1. The incidence of tuberculosis depends in part on the prevalence of a positive reaction to PPD. In general, if the incidence of a positive PPD skin reaction is low, there is a low incidence of active tuberculosis, without further new exposure. In a population with a large number of people who have a positive tuberculin reaction, the incidence of active

disease will be greater than in a population with a low prevalence of a reaction to this skin test antigen[5,7].

2. This is irrespective of the prevalence of infectious cases of tuberculosis in that population. That is, even if there are no infectious cases in a population, there will continue to be new active cases appearing in the previously infected individuals, even years after the infection occurred, and the frequency of new cases will reflect the skin test reactivity rate.

3. It has been shown that those factors which suppress immunity, for example, some drugs, certain diseases, or alcoholism, can destabilize latent tuberculosis. If this occurs in a population which has a high positive reaction to PPD, the incidence of active tuberculosis will also be high.

Since tuberculosis was a much more common problem 40 or 50 years ago, it is known that a positive reaction to PPD is much more common in older individuals[5,8] than in the population under 60 years of age. Since these older persons were alive when tuberculosis was common, they have had a greater opportunity to be infected and are at greater risk of developing clinical disease later in life. It has also been postulated that age, and the problems associated with increasing age, may also diminish the immune response to a variety of challenges[5,9].

As a result, the older individual who is more likely to have a positive PPD reaction than the general population can also, either because of ageing or the health problems associated with ageing, be much more likely to develop active tuberculosis.

CLINICAL DISEASE

The appearance of active tuberculosis in an older person is usually accompanied by the symptoms and signs usually seen in any age group. Malaise, fatigue, fever, night sweats, weight loss, productive cough, and haemoptysis may be some of the complaints expressed. The patient appears ill, may be cachectic, have inappropriate ADH (antidiuretic hormone) production, low serum sodium or chlorides, and debility.

It should be pointed out, however, that some of the symptoms of tuberculosis are a reflection of the patient's immune response to the disease. As a result, the person with blunted or absent immunity may be remarkably free of symptoms until they are desperately ill. This is evidenced by the effects of the not uncommon practice of giving steroid therapy to individuals who are very ill with tuberculosis to stabilize them until chemotherapy can become effective. Steroids in these cases will ameliorate the symptoms of fever and malaise, improve appetite, and in general suppress the symptoms of the disease[9,10].

Another complicating factor in the diagnosis of tuberculosis in the older person is the frequent presence of other chronic illness. Chronic bronchitis and emphysema, congestive heart failure, and carcinoma of the lung all mimic the symptoms and signs of tuberculosis; and these diseases are much more common in the older person than in other age groups[5]. The relative frequency of these disorders as compared to the increasing rarity of tuberculosis leads to a high index of suspicion for these other illnesses but complacency about a treatable infectious disease.

Tuberculosis is unfortunately often diagnosed at autopsy and may be ignored as a diagnostic possibility while repetitive, elaborate, expensive, and fruitless testing for other disorders is made[11,12].

The single most important factor for making the diagnosis of tuberculosis is to consider it as a possibility in the differential and to act on that suspicion[1,12].

Physical findings in tuberculosis can be minimal or absent but usually are those of râles, often in the posterior apical segment of the upper lobes, the superior segment of the lower lobes, with rhonchi, and occasionally the sound of air moving in a cavity – amphonic breathing. There may be dullness to percussion if there is a pleural effusion, pleural thickening, or a fibrotic or consolidated lung. The trachea, at least in advanced cases, may be deviated toward the side of the chest containing the disease.

The diagnosis and management of tuberculosis is heavily dependent on the laboratory findings, since the clinical features of the disorder are diverse, variable, and non-specific[2].

The chest X-ray, skin test, and examination of sputa for acid-fast bacilli are the critical laboratory tests when considering tuberculosis.

The tuberculin skin test, if positive, indicates prior exposure and infection with mycobacteria. The standard preparation, purified protein derivative (PPD), is neither pure nor does it contain only protein. It is partially purified when compared to old tuberculin (OT) which was previously used. At present, all PPD has added Tween® 80 to stabilize the antigen and prevent its adsorption on inert surfaces found in such items as needles and plastic syringes[7].

The acceptable practice is to apply the intermediate strength PPD (5 units) subcutaneously and observe the results 48 hours later. A positive test should be recorded by measuring the average diameter of induration. It should be pointed out, however, that a positive test can be read on the third or fourth day without significant loss of accuracy. A positive test conventionally is a reaction 10 mm in diameter or greater, but any induration is of interest and should be recorded and considered.

If the skin test to 5 units is negative, it is worthwhile to apply second strength PPD (250 units) since some individuals who are negative to 5 units will respond to 250 units as in severely ill individuals. The incidence of false-positive reactions are higher with second strength PPD, but that is clinically acceptable if the physician uses judgement[11].

The second strength should not be used initially since it can produce a severe local or even systemic reaction in some individuals.

The tine test, or its variants, are useful for public health work or as a part of routine screening for tuberculosis, as in a nursing home, but should not be relied upon where clinical disease is suspected.

Routine submission of sputa, or other body fluids, for acid-fast staining is a part of the diagnostic workup of a patient with suspected tuberculosis. It should be remembered that the sample size is small and the number of bacilli are few. This is particularly true in pleural or cerebral spinal fluid. As a result, concentration of the bacilli by appropriate means is useful; but even with the addition, it is not unusual to have active disease with negative smears.

Cultures for mycobacteria are much more effective in identifying the organisms and permit drug sensitivity testing. Unfortunately, 8–12 weeks may ensue before the organisms will be identified; and the clinician must, after obtaining them, be prepared to treat on the clinical grounds while awaiting cultures.

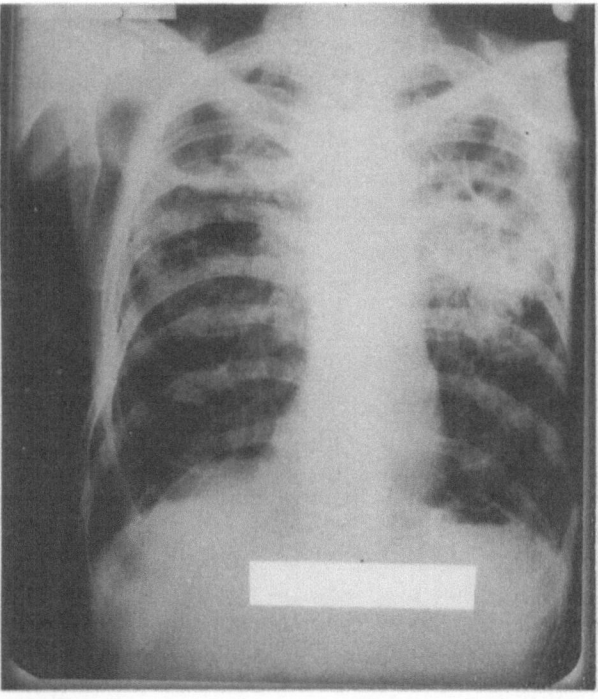

Figure 7.1   Well-advanced pulmonary tuberculosis, note bilateral fibrotic lesion with multiple large cavities and the area of alveolar spread in the left mid-lung field

In uncooperative patients, gastric aspirate obtained as a morning specimen after an overnight fast will provide organisms for culture. Smears of this material are not reliable because of false positives.

The chest X-ray findings in tuberculosis are usually a localized fibrotic cavitary infiltrate with a predilection for the apical posterior segment of the upper lobe or the superior segment of the lower lobe. While lesions outside these areas can occur, they are infrequent without simultaneous involvement of the classically involved segments (Figures 7.1 and 7.2). Areas of recent spread appear as an alveolar infiltrate, often of segmental or lobar distribution in dependent areas of the lung[13].

The X-ray differential diagnosis of tuberculosis is diverse, but the more common diseases which can mimic active pulmonary tuberculosis especially in older patients are pyogenic lung abscess, carcinoma of the lung with cavities, and the fungal diseases, especially histoplasmosis. Consideration of the clinical history together with further testing may be helpful in discriminating between tuberculosis and the rest of the differential diagnoses.

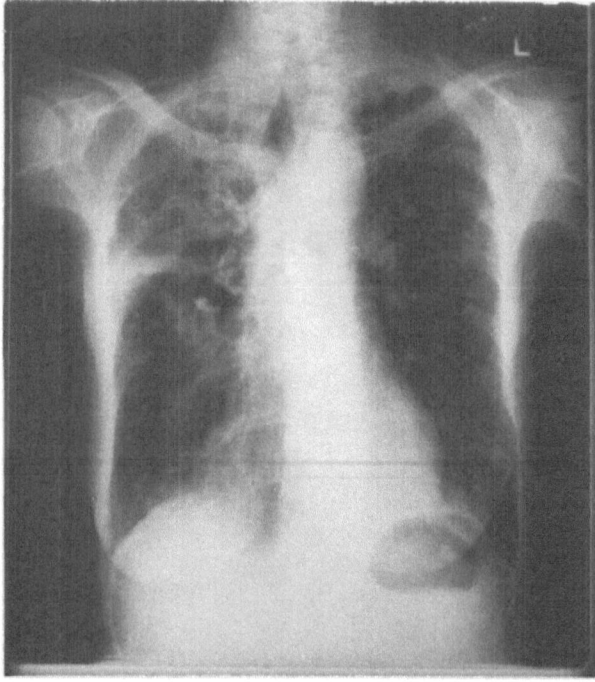

Figure 7.2 Chronic right upper lobe tuberculosis with upward retraction of the right hila, deviation of the trachea, with multiple cavities of the lung, pleural thickening, and hyperinflation of the right lower lobe, the left upper lobe is also involved with dense fibronodular infiltrates and apical pleural thickening

For example, lung abscess usually appears after an acute pneumonitis, is associated with a high temperature, and also often with a large volume of purulent sputa. As a routine, the fungal disorders should be eliminated by appropriate cultures and obtaining serological titres for histoplasmosis and coccidiomycosis. Skin testing with fungal antigens to rule out infection with specific fungi is sometimes useful in patients from geographic areas of high prevalence, but use of the skin test antigens may interfere with evaluation of fungal serology[14]. The diagnosis of North American blastomycosis is a rare and difficult problem because of the lack of specificity of its fungal serology, but it can be identified by culture.

Bronchoscopy in tuberculosis is usually unwarranted and may be hazardous if the anecdotal reports of post-bronchoscopy spread of disease are to be believed. Only when the preliminary evaluation for tuberculosis is negative should this valuable diagnostic procedure be considered. It should be remarked that reactivation of active pulmonary tuberculosis coincident with bronchogenic carcinoma can occur. In those instances where active tuberculosis has been identified and carcinoma of the lung is also suspected, the best course to follow is to initiate therapy for tuberculosis and after a suitable interval to allow a reduction in mycobacterial census and infectability, bronchoscopic evaluation can be obtained. That interval has not been established and the guidelines which have been advocated are not supported by acceptable data. It would seem reasonable that 1 month of therapy should greatly reduce infectiveness of patients and reduce the hazard to the personnel involved particularly in the view that cough will be suppressed by the narcotic which is used during evaluation of the lower airway.

Bronchoscopy should not be employed without consideration of the problems associated with its use and the fact that other methods are usually effective in establishing the diagnosis.

SIDE-EFFECTS OF ANTITUBERCULOUS DRUGS

Table 7.1 contains a summary of the major side-effects of the commonly employed antituberculous drugs[15]. In general, the commonly used antituberculous drugs are low in toxicity and have a good margin of safety.

Isoniazid

Isoniazid-induced hepatitis is a toxic reaction produced by direct damage to liver cells by the drug or its metabolites. It is usually mild and can be transient even if the drug is continued. Symptoms not unlike viral hepatitis occur, particularly malaise, anorexia, and, if severe, jaundice.

It has been clearly documented that the incidence of isoniazid hepatitis is age-related with an increasing incidence after the age of 40. In addition, there is some evidence that heavy consumption of alcohol predisposes to the problem. The problem can be serious on occasion, and deaths have been reported when the drug is continued despite serious liver damage. As a result, isoniazid therapy in the older patients should be followed more closely than in younger individuals and the patient and his family warned to stop the drug and consult the physician if symptoms of possible hepatitis occur. It has been advocated by some that monitoring of liver enzymes should be routinely done in older patients; but considering all the factors involved, this is probably not necessary unless there is pre-existing liver disease or other factors leading to more than usual insecurity about the patient. How often to obtain enzymes has not been settled, but it seems reasonable that 2 weeks after starting therapy, 1 month, and 2 months later seem reasonable intervals to obtain enzymes, although certainly the problem can appear any time after therapy is initiated. Mild elevation of enzymes indicates greater vigilance and more frequent testing but not necessarily stopping the drug. However, continued rise in enzymes mandates cessation of isoniazid therapy, and after the recovery of the patient it may be restarted with caution.

Table 7.1 Drugs commonly used to treat tuberculosis and their side-effects

Drug	Adult dosage (per day)	Major side-effects	Detection	Remarks
Isoniazid	300 mg	peripheral neuritis, hepatitis*, convulsions	liver enzymes	for neuritis, vitamin B₆ 25–50 mg as prophylaxis; hepatitis rare in young
Ethambutol	15 mg/kg	optic neuritis (very rare at 15 mg/kg)	visual acuity; red–green colour discrimination	ocular history and visual examination before use
Rifampicin	600mg	gastrointestinal disturbance, liver dysfunction, thrombocytopenia, and anticoagulation, rare renal damage, flu syndrome	SGOT / SGPT; bilirubin; BUN: creatinine	coloured urine occurs
Pyrazinamide	20–35 mg/kg (maximum 3g day)	gastrointestinal disturbance, hepatic dysfunction*, hyperuricaemia, photosensitivity	liver enzymes; uric acid	hepatitis is dose-related
Streptomycin	0.75–1.0g	otic and vestibular toxicity*, decreased hearing, vertigo, tinnitis	gross hearing; audiograms	cumulative ototoxicity*

* Age related

Rifampicin

Rifampicin, like isoniazid, is bacteriocidal but, unlike the latter, is an antibiotic with a fairly broad spectrum of antibacterial activity which has proved useful in other ways, for example, as prophylaxis for meningococcal meningitis. It is a powerful antituberculous agent probably equal to isoniazid and the combination of isoniazid and rifampicin is, at present, the mainstay of tuberculosis therapy. Its addition to the therapeutic armamentarium has allowed the significant shortening of the total length of therapy for tuberculosis which has been shown to be as effective as the longer periods of therapy used a decade ago.

Side-effects of rifampicin are uncommon. Hepatotoxicity, bone marrow suppression with anaemia, leukopenia, or thrombocytopenia can occur but are reversible if the drug is stopped. A flu-like syndrome has been reported with malaise, fever, chills, and myalgia. It is thought to be immune in nature, like the haematopoietic and hepatotoxic side-effects of this drug.

A potentially serious side-effect of rifampicin can occur because of its interaction with certain drugs metabolized by the liver. Rifampicin induces liver microsomal enzymes and starting or stopping the drug may alter the blood levels of other drugs such as the coumarin anticoagulants, some of the digitalis preparations, oral antihyperglycaemic drugs, corticosteroids, and oestrogenic hormones, all of which are frequently administered to older patients. As a result, these drugs should be administered with caution when rifampicin is used, and appropriate monitoring of their effects or their serum levels should be performed. In the case of digoxin and coumarin, the dose may have to be increased when therapy with rifampicin is started and reduced when the latter is discontinued.

Rifampicin also imparts an orange colouring to urine, and perspiration which can alarm patients but is of no significance.

Ethambutol

Ethambutol is a much less powerful chemotherapeutic agent than rifampicin or isoniazid. It can produce optic neuritis, but this is dose dependent and if the dose of 15mg/kg is used, this is rare. Ethambutol is a drug most often used during the initial phase of therapy where the number of mycobacteria is thought to be large, and it is usually continued for the first 60 days of treatment.

Pyrazinamide

Pyrazinamide is not widely used in developed countries for the therapy of tuberculosis. It is as potent, or even more potent, than isoniazid or rifampicin; but its use has been inhibited by its early reputation of producing serious liver cell damage which can be fatal. This latter problem is clearly dose-related and can be more frequent during prolonged therapy, in alcoholics, or in persons with prior liver disease.

Pyrazinamide can also induce hyperuricaemia, and it occasionally precipitates clinical gout, but this can be controlled by concomitant administration of a uric acid antimetabolite such as allopurinol, if needed. Occasionally, a photoreaction-related brownish discoloration of the skin occurs in patients on pyrazinamide but clears when therapy is stopped.

Streptomycin

Streptomycin is infrequently used in the treatment of tuberculosis. Like all aminoglycosides, it must be given by injection and this is costly and inconvenient. Since it can be given by injection, it can be used in individuals who cannot be given oral medication for any reason and was used occasionally for that reason. Since rifampicin by injection has become available, this useful indication has diminished in importance. It is still used in intermittent therapy and for therapy of infections with drug resistant organisms including *Mycobacterium intracellular aveum*.

The major side-effect of streptomycin is damage to the VIIIth cranial nerve with both auditory and vestibular symptoms. The incidence of this side-effect is total dose, age and renal function related. It is wise therefore to avoid the drug or reduce the dose in older or renal impaired persons. Indeed, its use in the elderly individuals is not recommended unless there is some clearly documented indication particularly in light of the availability of other less toxic agents.

Other Antituberculous Drugs

Other antituberculous drugs such as capreomycin, ethionomide, para-aminosalicylic acid, and cycloserine are rarely used to treat tuberculosis. The most frequent indication for their use is therapy of infections caused by organisms resistant to conventional antituberculous agents[16]. They should be used with caution in a well-planned programme using drug sensitivity data to establish a long-term strategy for providing adequate drug coverage using multiple agents. Single-agent therapy or poorly planned therapy leads only to further drug resistance and failure.

THERAPY OF ACTIVE TUBERCULOSIS IN THE ELDERLY

In general, therapy of tuberculosis is very effective and safe[15], but certain caveats must be observed when treatment is initiated in an older person. For example, renal excretion of drugs is more often impaired in this age group than in others. As a result, the dose of streptomycin, if used, must be adjusted. The frequency of hepatotoxicity of isoniazid has been clearly shown to be age-related[15].

Other problems related to therapy in the older person are more social and psychological in nature. Compliance with complicated therapeutic regimes may be less in the elderly than in others. Older people are frequently treated with several drugs for the chronic therapy of other non-tuberculous illnesses such as hypertension, heart failure, or Parkinson's disease. The addition of another group of drugs, in someone who may dislike drug-taking, who may be confused or who ascribes any new symptoms to medication may lead to non-compliance sufficient to impair effective treatment of tuberculosis.

There are certain basic rules that should guide the therapy of tuberculosis irrespective of age. Compliance with the drug programme is essential. The commonest cause of treatment failure is the patient not following the therapeutic programme provided by the physician. Alcoholism, mental disease, social disorganization, lack of adequate supervision, and family support have all been cited as causes of non-compliance.

It is essential that the physician, the public health support team, and the family of the patient co-operate to ensure that the patient is taking his drugs as prescribed and that any side-effects of those drugs are brought to the attention of the physician. In this context, this group must also ensure that the patient is aware of and follows the rules to prevent dissemination of his disease to others. Since effective chemotherapy is the single most important factor in reducing and eliminating the infectiousness of tuberculosis, adequate chemotherapy, when complied with, is the keystone of controlling the spread of this disorder[17,18.]

The decision to start therapy should not await clinical proof of the disorder such as a positive smear of the sputum for acid-fast bacilli or cultural evidence for mycobacteria. The latter can often take months and will be irrelevant in certain forms of the disorder such as widespread disease or in meningitis. The clinician must be prepared to treat on the basis of clinical judgement where the symptoms and chest X-ray are compatible with the disease while containing evaluation of the patient. An X-ray compatible with active tuberculosis with a positive skin test with PPD is a powerful argument not to delay therapy. It is almost always better to start therapy and later stop than to wait until the disease has progressed and the staff exposed to the disease. Chemotherapy will not interfere with a diagnostic workup, except in genitourinary tuberculosis.

When considering chemotherapy, the physician must attempt to rule out the possibility of drug-resistant organisms, such as strains of *M. tuberculosis* which usually occur because of inadequate previous chemotherapy. Primary drug resistance as opposed to induced resistance is rare and usually suggests an atypical mycobacterial infection. Drug resistance may be a more common problem in patients who have lived in developing countries, since this complication is more common in patients from these areas than in the industrialized nations[19, 20].

Initial isolates of mycobacteria should be routinely tested for drug sensitivity; and if the patient who is on therapy does not do well, has a recurrence, or has been erratic in taking medications, the sputa should be recultured for mycobacteria; and if organisms are found, they should be rechecked for sensitivity[16].

THEORY OF MULTIPLE DRUGS IN TUBERCULOSIS

Any of the three most potent antituberculous drugs, isoniazid, rifampicin, and pyrazinamide, given alone, can produce clinical improvement in active tuberculosis. Unfortunately, this favourable course is often only temporary; and within some months, drug-resistant organisms will appear in the sputa and the clinical symptoms of the disease re-emerge.

Drug resistance in mycobacteria is an independent event for the drug in each organism. If one bacteria in 10^5 organisms is resistant to isoniazid and one in 10^4 is resistant to streptomycin, then the chances of encountering an isoniazid – streptomycin-resistant organism is only one in 10^9 bacteria, a very large number. If these two drugs were given, theoretically this number, 10^9, would exceed the numbers of mycobacteria present; and this therapy, if given for a sufficient period of time, should be successful. As a matter of fact, this theoretical prediction has been shown to be true by accumulated clinical experiences[17, 21].

Where the numbers of mycobacteria are limited, as in pleuritis or in tuberculous meningitis, the clinical response to two drugs, isoniazid and ethambutol, the latter a relatively weak drug, can have a satisfactory outcome. Even in cavitary pulmonary tuberculosis where there are more bacilli than in pleuritis, isoniazid and ethambutol can be effective. To achieve this, however, the drugs must be given for a period of time sufficient to kill most of the mycobacteria, usually 18 months to 2 years. This was standard therapy for years.

Substituting another first-line bacteriocidal drug of greater potency such as rifampicin may influence outcome slightly in a 2-year programme, usually when there are very large number of organisms; but the major advantage of adding a second first-line drug such as rifampicin has been to allow a reduction of the length of therapy while still preserving an acceptable rate of recurrence. Therapy for pulmonary tuberculosis using two first-line drugs such as isoniazid and rifampicin can be given for 1 year or less with a satisfactory outcome except in the most far advanced disease. If three first-line drugs are used, even 6 months' therapy with a favourable outcome may be possible[22-24].

If these concepts are put into perspective, then it can be observed that the cost and perhaps the incidence of side-effects of the additional drugs in short-course chemotherapy can be balanced against the risks of a longer period of therapy with other drugs, with the possibility of the patient discontinuing his drugs or being lost to follow-up. In the stable person with substantial roots in the community, this may be less important compared with alcoholics, transients, or unmotivated individuals. As a result, the drugs are employed for 9–12 months, have become standard care, and are always used except where drug-resistant organisms are suspected, toxicity has occurred, or where large caseous lesions are treated, as in abscesses.

INITIAL DRUG THERAPY

In previously untreated tuberculosis, a programme using isoniazid and rifampicin (Table 7.2) is sufficient in most instances. This combination is usually free of side-effects, relatively simple, and effective. Patient tolerance is good; and since duration of therapy is usually 9 months to 1 year, compliance is good. If there is very extensive disease involving large numbers of mycobacteria, or the disease is extrapulmonary, ethambutol should also be administered for the first 60 days of treatment[17, 22, 25].

Table 7.2 Therapy of pulmonary tuberculosis in adults

Isoniazid	300 mg/day as a single daily dose
Rifampicin	600 mg/day as a single daily dose
Ethambutol	15 mg/kg/day for the first 60 days (optional)

Therapy of osseous, renal, lymph node, and genital tuberculosis sometimes requires therapy for 1 year to 18 months. Lastly, miliary and meningeal infections or a tuberculous pleural effusion can be treated using conventional therapy, since the number of organisms are relatively few and two drugs for 9 months will usually be adequate[17, 22].

Progress during therapy can be noted by observing defervescence, improved appetite and well-being, weight gain, and reduced cough. Improvement on chest X-ray may not occur for several months. When it occurs, it includes clearing of infiltrates and the closure of small or medium-sized cavities. Residual cavitation and considerable post-infection scarring of the lung is not uncommon, particularly if the individual has extensive disease. These unfavourable changes will persist despite adequate therapy and there may be areas of residual bronchiectasis. Because of the location of these bronchial changes, the patient is usually asymptomatic despite the persistent damage to the bronchi.

The primary considerations in choosing a therapeutic regimen depend on an absence of a history of previous therapy and a judgement that the patient can be expected to be reasonably co-operative and take his medications regularly.

Total duration of therapy in pulmonary tuberculosis is 9 months except in those instances in which there is extensive disease (such as multiple lobe involvement, numerous cavities). In those instances, it is suggested that 1 year of chemotherapy be used. This seems reasonable, since the possibility of recurrence is greater in these individuals, but data to support this position is not available.

Intermittent therapy appears to be as effective as conventional daily treatment[22], but probably has no place in the routine therapy of tuberculosis since effective therapy using daily drugs has become the standard against which other programmes of treatment must be judged. The intermittent programme has advantages in the treatment of disease in those patients who cannot or will not follow a routine programme. An intermittent programme given to that group of patients requires strict supervised administration of the drugs, close monitoring of effectiveness, and the involvement of sufficient medical and social services to maintain contact and supervision of the patients offered this form of treatment. It is of necessity more expensive and will be more intrusive in their lives than conventional programmes.

HOSPITALIZATION

Hospital care is not essential but should be offered on the basis of need. Severely ill patients, patients with other medical problems or haemoptysis, and those who have liver or renal disease, should probably be hospitalized, at least until they are stabilized.

If the patient is hospitalized, isolation in a room fitted with a negative pressure ventilation system is necessary[26]. This usually consists of an exhaust fan providing a flow of air from the room to the outside. Hospital personnel in contact with the patient do not require gowns, and the mask most commonly offered to hospital personnel only provides a false sense of security. Since infectious droplets are generated by coughing, the patient should be instructed to cough into a disposable tissue, which can be burned. If the patient is to be transported, a face mask on the patient will probably be of value. Decontamination of the room after discharge consists of airing the room for 12 hours, wiping the surface of the furniture, and mopping the floor. If it is remembered that only by the inhalation of infectious droplets do hospital personnel become infected, it can be seen that much of the isolation ritual used in the past was unnecessary.

Most hospital personnel who become infected with mycobacteria do so by caring for patients with unrecognized and untreated disease.

Patients with tuberculosis who are on ventilators are not infectious if there is an exhaust filter fitted on the machine. During suctioning of the patient on a ventilator, when the system is opened, the person involved should be prepared to shield the tube if the patient coughs, using a disposable tissue. Risk during this procedure should be low because of the size of the particles generated.

STEROIDS IN THE THERAPY OF TUBERCULOSIS

In the desperately ill individual who has extensive pulmonary tuberculosis, or in instances of meningeal tuberculosis, administration of corticosteroids, such as prednisone, may be lifesaving. Because many of the symptoms of tuberculosis are part of the immune reaction to the disease, malaise, poor appetite, fever, and other symptoms can be suppressed while awaiting the effect of chemotherapy. The usual dose is 40–60 mg of prednisone (or equivalent) until the patient is stabilized and then the dose is slowly reduced over a period of several weeks.

While meningeal tuberculosis is a rare event in the elderly, it should be pointed out that steroids are widely used to ameliorate the scarring which occurs at the base of the brain and results in internal hydrocephalus and damage to the cranial nerves.

CONTACTS OF TUBERCULOUS PATIENTS

The close contacts of patients with active pulmonary tuberculosis must be skin tested. Examples of close contacts are members of their household, co-workers in the immediate vicinity, and those who might also be confined with the source case in the same room for significant periods of time. Reactors should be evaluated for clinical disease and prophylaxis offered if appropriate.

TUBERCULOSIS IN THE NURSING HOME

Active tuberculosis is a relatively common problem in nursing homes. The coincidence of debility and a relatively high rate of skin test reactivity to the purified protein derivative (PPD) of *M. tuberculosis* among this population leads to a high risk of reactivation of latent infection. Symptoms that develop in nursing home patients are often overlooked among the many medical problems of the individuals who reside in these facilities. As a result, physicians who care for these patients must be alert for the possibility of active tuberculosis and the facility must have an ongoing control programme for tuberculosis[1].

The control of tuberculosis in a nursing home is simple if a preventive programme is implemented. All patients should have PPD skin tests on admission, and those with positive reactions should have a chest film. Those with positive skin tests must be identified as special risks and have biannual chest X-rays. Those with abnormal films, either on admission or later, should be evaluated with appropriate diagnostic studies.

PROPHYLAXIS OF TUBERCULOSIS

It has been established that 1 year of isoniazid therapy without a companion antituberculous drug will prevent clinical active disease in certain high-risk groups (Table 7.3). In general, these are individuals who have been recently infected, as demonstrated by conversion of their PPD skin test from negative to positive, individuals with positive skin tests who have their immunity suppressed, or individuals exposed to tuberculosis in an uncontrolled situation[27].

Isoniazid therapy is also used to cover individuals with a history of a positive skin test on immunosuppressive therapy. It should also be noted that low dose steroid therapy is probably not immunosuppressive in the context of this discussion[10].

Table 7.3 Indications for isoniazid prophylaxis

1. Individuals known to have converted their skin test within the previous 2 years.
2. Household contacts of cases of infectious tuberculosis during evaluation of their status or as long as the contact persists.
3. Patients who have a positive skin test and who will receive chronic immunosupressive therapy.
4. Patients who have had active tuberculosis in the past and who have not received a satisfactory course of chemotherapy; these are usually older persons with a history of bed rest or collapse therapy in the prechemotherapy era.
5. Persons with a positive skin test who are under 35 years of age.

CONTROL OF INFECTION

The solution to the problem of infectiousness of tuberculosis is prompt and effective chemotherapy[27]. If the patient is started on effective drugs, he is usually non-infectious within a few weeks[26]. Since the most infectious period is usually the time just before the disease is diagnosed, once chemotherapy is begun they are much less of a risk than before therapy[28]. If the patient can go home and is reliable, this is a most suitable course to follow, remembering to deal appropriately with the family contacts.

SUMMARY

Tuberculosis can be a serious problem in the elderly. The higher than usual incidence of infection with mycobacteria, often remotely, in this group of individuals coupled with other chronic illness and debility leads to a high incidence of clinical disease, when compared to younger age groups.

Diagnosis of active disease requires a high index of suspicion by the physician caring for the older person, with prompt evaluation for the disease when the diagnosis is suspected. Evaluation is simple, employing the PPD skin test, appropriate X-rays, and submission of appropriate body fluids for bacteriological examination, including smears and cultures.

Treatment in suspected cases should not await bacteriological confirmation. A programme of isoniazid and rifampicin is relatively safe, effective, will control infectiousness, and results in cure of the disorder.

References

1. Kasik, J. E. and Schuldt, S. (1977). Why tuberculosis is still a problem in the aged. *Geriatrics*, **32,** 63–72
2. Myers, J. A. (1965). The natural history of tuberculosis in the human body. *J. Am. Med. Assoc.*, **194,** 184–90
3. Stead, W. W. (1967). Pathogenesis of a first episode of chronic pulmonary tuberculosis in man: recrudecence of residuals of primary infection or exogenous reinfection. *Am. Rev. Resp. Dis.*, **95,** 729–34
4. Rich, A. R. (1951). *The Pathogenesis of Tuberculosis*. 2nd Ed., p. 882. (Springfield, Ill.: C. C. Thomas)
5. Stead, W. W. (1965). The pathogenesis of tuberculosis among older persons. *Am. Rev. Resp. Dis.*, **91,** 811–17
6. Berger, H. W. and Mejia, E. (1973). Tuberculous pleurisy. *Chest*, **63,** 88–92
7. Snider, D. E. (1982). The tuberculin skin test. *Am. Rev. Resp. Dis.*, **125,** (2), 108–18
8. Lowell, A. M. (1969). *Tuberculosis: 1: Morbidity and Mortality and Its Control*. Vital Health Statistics Monograph. American Public Health Association. (Cambridge, Mass.: Harvard University Press)
9. Collins, F. M. (1982). The immunity of tuberculosis. *Am. Rev. Resp. Dis.*, **125,** (2), 42–9
10. Sahn, S. A. and Lakshminarayan, S. (1976). Tuberculosis after corticosteroid therapy. *Chest*, **70,** 195–200
11. Edlin, G. P. (1978). Active tuberculosis unrecognized until necropsy. *Lancet*, **1,** 650–2
12. Bobrowitz, I. D. (1982). Active tuberculosis undiagnosed until autopsy. *Am. J. Med.*, **72,** 650–8
13. Miller, W. T. and MacGregor, R. R. (1978). Tuberculosis: frequency of unusual radiographic findings. *Am. J. Roentgenol.*, **130,** 867–5
14. Terry, P. B., Rosenow, E. C. and Roberts, G. D. (1978). False positive complement-fixation serology in histoplasmosis, a retrospective study. *J. Am. Med. Assoc.*, **239,** 2453–6
15. Gerling, D. J. (1982). Adverse effect of antituberculous drugs. *Drugs*, **23,** 56–74
16. Guernsey, B. G., Alexander, M. R. (1978). Tuberculosis: review of treatment failure, relapse and drug resistance. *Am. J. Hosp. Pharmacol.*, **35,** 690–8

17. Byrd, R. B., Kaplan, P. D. and Gracey, D. R. (1974). Treatment of pulmonary tuberculosis, critical review. *Chest*, **66**, 560–7
18. Addington, W. W. (1979). The treatment of pulmonary tuberculosis, current options. *Arch: Intern. Med.*, **139**, 1391–5
19. (1983). Primary resistance to antituberculous drugs – United States. MMWR, **32**, 516–518
20. Livengood, J. R., Sigler, T. G., Foster, L. R., Bobst, J. G. and Snider, D. E. (1985). Isoniazid-resistant tuberculosis, a community outbreak and a report of rifampicin prophylaxis failure. *J. Am. Med. Assoc.*, **253**, 2847–2849
21. Canetti, G. (1964). Host factors and chemotherapy of tuberculosis. *Chemotherapy of Tuberculosis*. (London: Butterworths)
22. Stead, W. W. and Dutt, A. K. (1981). What's new in tuberculosis. *Am. J. Med.*, **71**, 1–4
23. Short course chemotherapy in pulmonary tuberculosis, a controlled trial by the British Thoracic and Tuberculosis Association (1976). *Lancet*, **2**, 1102–5
24. Mehrotta, J. L. Goutam, K. D., Chaube, C. K. and Mesra, J. B. (1979). Semi-supervised clinical trial of nine months chemotherapy without rifampicin in pulmonary tuberculosis. *Bull. Int. Union Tuberc.*, **54**, 9–21
25. Dutt, A. K. and Stead, W. W. (1980). Chemotherapy of tuberculosis for the 1980's. *Lancet*, **1**, 243–52
26. Riley, F. L., Mills, C. C. and O'Grady, F. (1962). Infectiousness of air from a tuberculosis ward. *Am. Rev. Respir. Dis.*, **85**, 511–25
27. Leff, A. L. and Geppert, E. F. (1979). Public health aspects of pulmonary tuberculosis, infectiousness, epidemiology, risk factor classification, and preventive therapy. *Arch. Intern. Med.*, **139**, 1405–9
28. Gunnels, J. J., Bates, J. H. and Sevindoll, H. (1974). Infectivity of sputum positive tuberculous patients on chemotherapy. *Am. Res. Respir. Dis.*, **109**, 323–30

8

Bone and Joint Infections

M. J. CLARKE-WILLIAMS

INTRODUCTION

Infections of the bones and joints are by no means the commonest infections that occur in the elderly. They are therefore ones that are easily forgotten in the diagnosis of the toxic older patient. The symptoms of osteomyelitis or pyogenic arthritis are vague and may mimic the 'aches and pains' often experienced by any ageing person. The signs too are often difficult to differentiate from the limitation of movement of the joints expected in older people. For their diagnosis to be made, the possibility of osteomyelitis and pyogenic arthritis must be borne in mind.

The incidence of osteomyelitis depends upon its cause. Where the infection is blood-borne there is a bimodal distribution with one peak in childhood and around puberty when the long bones only are affected. The second peak occurs between 50 years and 70 years when both long bones and vertebrae are affected. The incidence of haematogenous osteomyelitis has been increasing during recent years, although fortunately the mortality has been decreasing. Osteomyelitis due to contiguous spread and vascular insufficiency has a peak of incidence between 50 years and 70 years.

With the increasing proportion of the elderly, indeed of the very elderly, in the community with many long-standing disabilities, the incidence of bone and joint infections is likely to increase, particularly as the elderly are most subject to the predisposing factors of bone and joint trauma, and orthopaedic surgery.

Acute infections are usually swiftly dealt with by the wide range of antibiotics now available, but chronic infections are often hard to eradicate.

143

PATHOLOGY OF OSTEOMYELITIS

Osteomyelitis is the inflammation of bone due to a pyogenic organism. It may be localized or it may spread through the bone to involve the marrow, cancellous tissue, the cortex and the periosteum. In acute infections there is destruction of bone with formation of a sequestrum, due to the necrosis of cancellous tissue, following impairment of the blood supply. Chronic infections are associated, however, with sclerosis of bone. Periosteal involvement with abscess formation is less common in the elderly due to the firm attachment of the periosteum and the reduction in periosteal osteoblastic activity.

There are three possible courses that the infection may take. When the patient's resistance is good, the bone infection will be contained and then eradicated before any suppuration can occur. Where the infecting organism is more virulent a chronic localized focus of suppuration – a Brodie's abscess – may be formed. Alternatively, in patients with impaired resistance, a virulent infection may result in suppuration with death of bone, the formation of a sequestrum and of an envelope of new bone around the necrotic tissue producing an involucrum.

Three mechanisms are involved in the production of osteomyelitis. In one-half of cases there is contiguous spread from adjacent structures. In one-third of cases there is peripheral vascular disease. In the remaining one-fifth only is haematogenous spread responsible, perhaps because of the early use of antibiotics[1]. Despite its being the cause in a minority of cases, haematogenous spread is the most commonly discussed because it raises many problems. Why should one bone be more susceptible to attack than another? Why should a hip prosthesis become the site of an infection many years after the original operation? Why are the lumbar vertebrae attacked more often than the thoracic vertebrae, and the cervical vertebrae least often? With the relatively higher incidence of septicaemia in the elderly why are the bones so infrequently infected? Trauma to the bone is usually cited as the cause of these features but it remains a puzzle that mild or trivial trauma can precipitate osteomyelitis. The diagnosis may easily be overlooked if the site of the infection is no longer apparent and the trauma so long ago that it has been forgotten.

The excellent blood supply to the growth areas of bone such as the metaphysis, helps to explain why that part of the bone is attacked for preference. Once it is established, infection may be difficult to eradicate. The capillary loops in the metaphysis do not contain active phagocytosing lining cells. The blood flow in the loops is sluggish, and obstruction to the flow in them by inflammatory oedema could result in small areas of avascular necrosis[1].

The way in which blood-borne infections are carried to the vertebrae has been investigated[2]. It appears most likely that the infection is carried by the arteries to the metaphyseal region of the vertebrae where there is a rich blood supply via the nutrient arteries. It seems less likely that the infection is spread via the pelvic venous plexi. One of the earliest degenerations of ageing involves the intervertebral discs which lose their vasculature early and their nutrition is maintained by diffusion only. Usually the infection starts in the metaphysis of the vertebrae and spreads to the disc which is destroyed. This allows the spread of the infection to the adjacent vertebra with the provocation of vertebral collapse.

PATHOLOGY OF PYOGENIC ARTHRITIS

Pyogenic arthritis is the inflammation of a joint due to pyogenic organisms. The response of the joint depends upon the virulence of the invading organism, but it will involve the exudation of fluid into the synovial cavity. There are three main forms of response. There is the serous effusion where the joint is distended with clear fluid. This may subside without any further trouble. Where the inflamed synovial membrane becomes congested and thickened there is a serofibrinous exudate which contains polymorphonuclear leukocytes and large mononuclear cells. There will also be some inflammation of the periarticular tissues. In the most severe form of infection of a joint the effusion is frankly purulent and contains large numbers of polymorphonuclear leukocytes, bacteria, red blood corpuscles and fibrin. In the capsule and synovial membrane, which are engorged and infiltrated by leukocytes, there may be small areas of focal necrosis. The destruction spreads to the articular cartilage and the bone may be exposed leading to secondary osteomyelitis. Perforation of the capsule may occur with the formation of a periarticular abscess.

There are several routes by which the infection may reach the joint. It may occur during an acute infectious disease by haematogenous spread. Alternatively it may be secondary to an infection extending from an inflamed bone or from a compound fracture. Infection may also be directly implanted into a joint through a puncture wound.

BACTERIOLOGY OF OSTEOMYELITIS AND PYOGENIC ARTHRITIS

The organism that most commonly causes both osteomyelitis and pyogenic arthritis is *Staphylococcus pyogenes aureus,* which is a normal inhabitant of the human skin. In the haematogenous type of infection its incidence however has fallen from about 80–90% to 50–60% of cases[1]. However, it remains the most common infection in those cases due to contiguous spread and vascular insufficiency.

A variety of other organisms may be found. If the infection is due to *Staphylococcus albus* the symptoms are less acute. Fortunately β-haemolytic streptococci are less often responsible but are likely to produce multiple lesions. Both bones and joints may be infected by the tubercle bacillus, which as a rule spreads from an infection in the lung or elsewhere. The anterior border of a vertebra is often the site of tuberculous osteomyelitis, with spread to the intervertebral disc and the adjacent vertebra (Figure 8.1).

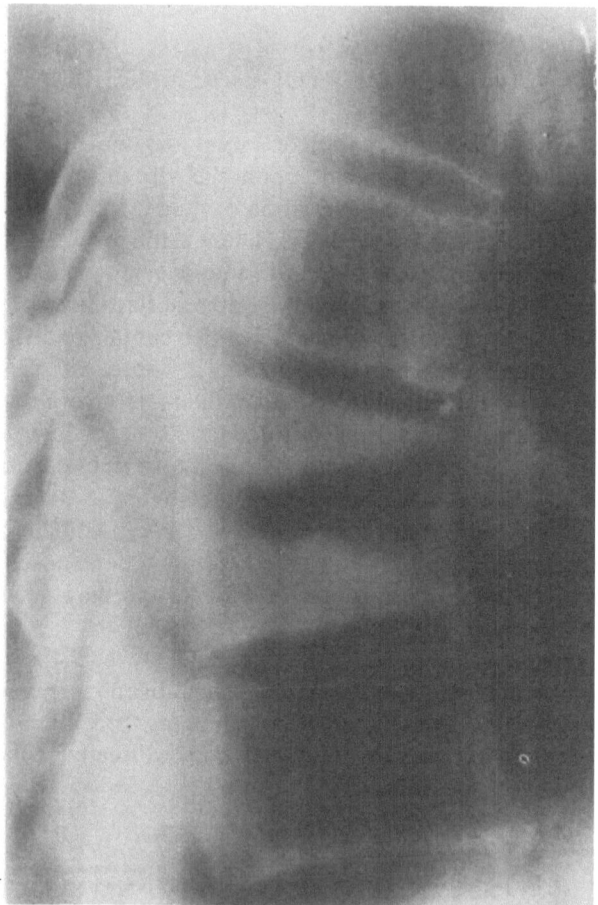

Figure 8.1 Tuberculosis of vertebral bodies with anterior collapse

Less common causes are *Escherichia coli,* and *Clostridium welchii,* which may be found in the wound following a compound fracture. Pneumococci, meningococci and gonococci may occasionally be found, as may typhoid bacilli, which infect vertebral bodies, ribs and may cause a pyogenic arthritis. A rare cause of infection in joint arthroplasties is an anaerobic organism like *Proprionibacterium acnes*[3]. If bone is involved from a septic wound, an ulcer or a pressure sore, the infection is likely to be due to a mixture of organisms.

Bacterial arthritis is usually due to haematogenous spread from a distant site of infection. Bruises, excoriations and small abrasions of the skin are very common in the elderly, whose skin is less supple than in the young and forms a less effective barrier to infection. Other sources of haematogenous bacterial spread are the oropharynx, nasal sinuses, middle ear, and the lung. The urogenital tract and the pelvic organs such as the colon are also sources.

PREDISPOSING FACTORS

The main predisposing cause for osteomyelitis in the elderly is trauma, which may be accidental or surgical. Accidental trauma may be surprisingly slight and may have occurred a great number of years ago, leaving an injury in which the infection subsequently settles. Pressure trauma can result from wearing tight shoes, which can cause an adventitious bursa to develop over the prominent head of the first metatarsal bone. Such a bunion may suppurate and ulcerate with the infection spreading to the underlying bone and the first metatarsophalangeal joint (Figure 8.2).

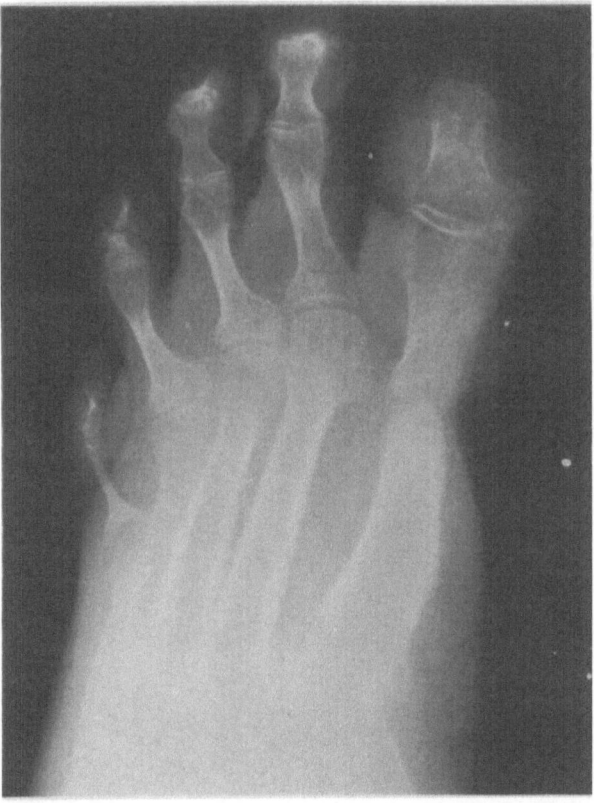

Figure 8.2 Destruction of the first metacarpophalangeal joint underlying a bunion

Surgical Trauma

Surgical trauma occurs in the form of joint replacements and the operative repair of fractures with prostheses or with plates and screws. Fractures of the neck of the femur are very common indeed in older people, particularly women, and the treatment of choice is by arthroplasty with the insertion of a prosthesis. Osteoarthritis of the hips and knees occurs frequently in the elderly and may be treated by total hip replacement or knee replacement. Fortunately less than half of 1% of patients who have had hip replacements, and less than 1% of those who have had knee replacements, develop subsequent infections. When an infection does develop at any time thereafter, it may result from contamination of the site during the operation or from haematogenous spread from a source of infection elsewhere in the body. At the site of the operation there is osteolysis, as the body tries to sequestrate the infected bony tissue and the implant which leads to loosening of the prosthesis and consequent instability of the joint (Figure 8.3).

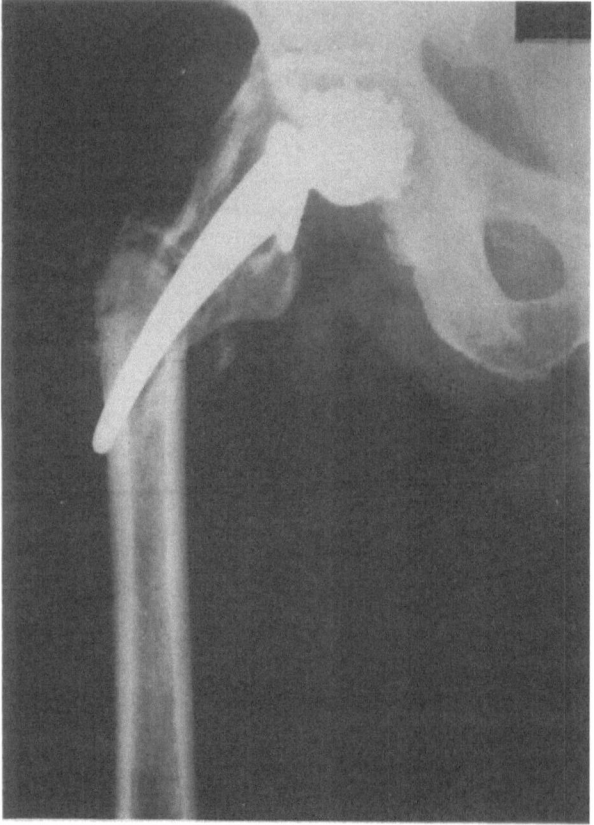

Figure 8.3 Osteomyelitis of the femur after hip replacement

Peripheral Vascular Disease

Elderly people frequently suffer from peripheral vascular disease – another predisposing factor. Arterial insufficiency occurs particularly in those who have been heavy cigarette smokers and in those with diabetes mellitus. If ischaemia leads to ulceration or moist gangrene there is a danger of the underlying bone developing osteomyelitis by direct extension of the infection. The small bones of the toes and feet are most often involved, so that patients complain of long-established ulcers on the feet which fail to heal. In many, unfortunately, the ischaemia may be of such severity that an amputation is required. When the amputation is a distal one the wound is often very difficult to heal. Before the Burgess long posterior flap was used, below-knee amputations were difficult to heal because of the inadequacy of the supply from the geniculate arteries. The sawn end of the bone is easily infected from such an unhealed wound, even if the marrow cavity is packed with bone chips. Above-knee amputations are usually much swifter to heal, but may be difficult even when a myoplastic technique is used (Figures 8.4 and 8.5). Sometimes, long after the amputation, due to the shrinkage of the musculature of the stump, the end of the bone causes ulceration of the overlying skin due to pressure below the skin. Osteomyelitis of the bone from these causes will necessitate a reamputation and reconstruction of the stump.

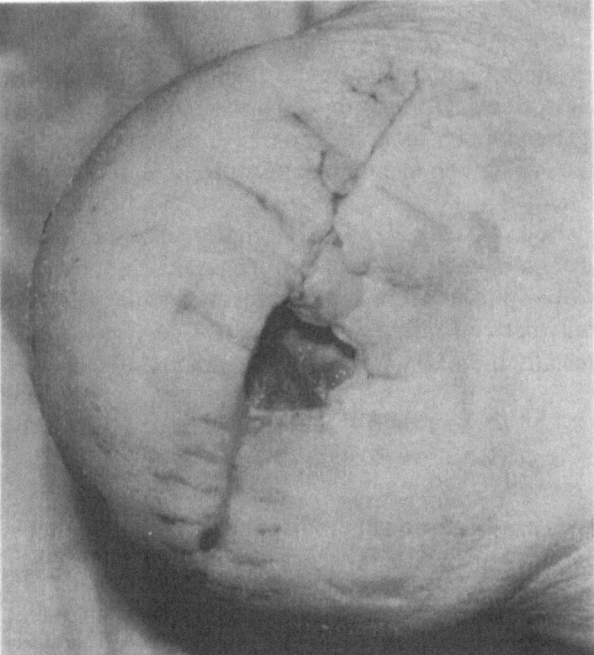

Figure 8.4 A chronic ulcer in an above-knee amputation scar

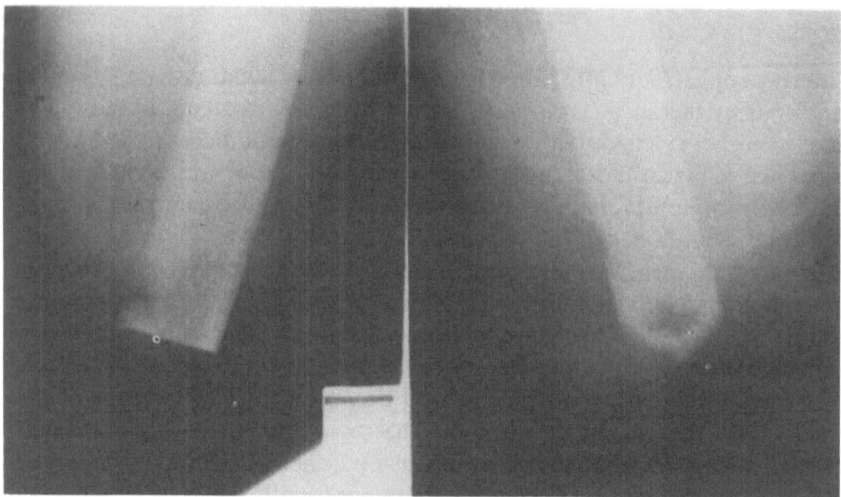

Figure 8.5   Osteomyelitis of the stump of the femur after amputation

Skin Ulceration

Skin ulceration of the calves is frequently seen, particularly in elderly women. This is caused by venous stasis, in part due to the patient sitting for long periods with her legs dependent and the consequent diminution of venous return, due to lack of muscular massage of the deep veins. Such ulceration is notoriously difficult to heal and keep healed. These ulcers are less frequently a cause of osteomyelitis of the underlying tibia than they are a source of infection for the haematogenous production of a pyogenic arthritis.

In diabetes mellitus there is disease of the small vessels and this may be accompanied by a sensory neuropathy. Together they predispose to the development of trophic ulcers of the feet that are again very slow to heal. It is very important that chiropody should be done very carefully on diabetic patients, especially the paring away of callosities.

Pressure Sores

Any patient who has enforced immobility due to disease or after surgery is at risk and may develop pressure sores. In particular, patients who have severe osteoarthritis or rheumatoid arthritis, or after orthopaedic operations, are liable to ulcerate over bony prominences such as the sacrum, superior iliac spines, ischial tuberosities, ankles or heels. If these pressure sores become chronically infected the underlying bone is in danger of developing osteomyelitis. This is particularly true when the sore develops a thick slough, which is bound down to the deeper structures by fibrous bands, in the interstices of which are pockets of infection. It is fortunate that due to the poor local blood supply haematogenous spread from these sores is unusual. The calcaneum under a heel sore however is vulnerable to a low grade osteomyelitis.

Rheumatoid arthritis is a common chronic condition in the elderly and some 10% of these patients have low grade sepsis in the knees. Any condition that diminishes the patient's resistance to an infection is also a predisposing factor. Examples include poor general nutrition, a malignant disease or other long-standing illness, or prolonged use of corticosteroids, cytotoxic drugs or radiotherapy.

CLINICAL PRESENTATION AND DIAGNOSIS

Both osteomyelitis and pyogenic arthritis when well established will have the classical four signs of inflammation – rubor, calor, tumor and dolor. The diagnosis of both should, however, be considered at a much earlier stage than this. The early symptoms are unfortunately rather vague with the older patient who fails to thrive. This may be ascribed to the patient's age, which is most unwise. The possibility of infection of a bone or joint should be considered in such cases. The patient's temperature is seldom much raised. Clues to the diagnosis may be the presence of chronic ulceration, or a discharging sinus. There may be a history of a fractured hip, with replacement, and a recent deterioration in the function of the joint. Patients with long bone involvement are more likely to have a low grade pyrexia than those where a vertebra is involved[4]. The sudden onset of pyrexia and a toxic state is less commonly seen in haematogenous osteomyelitis than previously[5]. Patients with vertebral osteomyelitis may complain of the recent onset of localized pain in the back, which may be worse on straining. There is seldom any root radiation, but the bone may be tender on percussion. Later signs of meningitis or cord compression may develop.

Pyogenic arthritis will present with a decreased range of movement in the affected joint and pain on movement. The joint may have clear signs of an effusion, which should always be aspirated and a biopsy taken if possible. Some 90% of cases have only one joint affected, usually the knee in half of all cases of pyogenic arthritis. There may be a leukocytosis of up to 200 000 in the purulent synovial fluid.

Chronic osteomyelitis can have several sequelae. Thus some patients with chronic bone infections, resistant to all forms of conservative treatment may develop signs of amyloidosis in the spleen, liver, kidney or adrenal glands. However, this complication occurs less often than in the past. Bone infection which has been present for many years may lead to the development of an epidermoid carcinoma, which may be found on the tibia or the femur.

The patient may have signs of peripheral vascular disease and, if he has diabetes mellitus, there may be the complications of retinopathy, nephropathy or neuropathy.

Routine blood tests may be unhelpful because the haemoglobin, white blood count and erythrocyte sedimentation rate (ESR) may be normal. Sometimes there is a leukocytosis of up to 16 000 and the ESR may be high. Biochemistry may show a raised alkaline phosphatase.

Bacteriological diagnosis is most important and organisms may be obtained from wound swabs, aspiration of synovial fluid or from bone biopsy. Blood cultures can be helpful but are negative in 50% of cases of vertebral osteomyelitis.

Radiology is very useful in diagnosis – soft tissue swelling and periosteal elevation are seen initially with lytic lesions becoming evident only after some weeks. Sclerotic lesions take several months to develop. Because of this it is wise to X-ray the bones again later if clinical suspicion remains.

Where vertebral osteomyelitis is due to tuberculous infection an early sign on X-ray is the herniation of the nucleus pulposus through the vertebral end plate into the trabecular bone of the vertebral body, with diminution of the joint space. Later the anterior border of the vertebra collapses producing an angular kyphosis. One-third of these patients develop signs of cord compression and even a paraplegia. In a minority of cases an X-ray of the chest shows tuberculous infection.

Unfortunately isotope bone scans are not very helpful since they do not distinguish between simple trauma, osteomyelitis or even a neoplasm.

Because vague complaints of pains in the bones or joints are common in the elderly, it is important to consider osteomyelitis or pyogenic arthritis when the general condition of the patient is worse than one might have expected.

TREATMENT

There is a significant increase both in the morbidity and in the mortality associated with delay in treatment of osteomyelitis or pyogenic arthritis in the elderly. The recognition of the condition may take a few weeks to many months or even a year. The treatment will, of course, depend not only on the precipitating cause but also on the causative organism. Antibiotics play an important part, but other measures are required as well.

Where osteomyelitis follows upon trauma or a surgical operation all the dead bone and the infected tissues must be removed. Surgery must also be considered for patients with severe complications such as cord compression, or where medical treatment has failed in those with peripheral vascular disease.

Antibiotics will be given according to the sensitivity of the causative organism. In the initial stages of the illness they may need to be given by intravenous or intramuscular injection and later by mouth. Courses of antibiotic treatment should be for a minimum of 3 months, or longer in the cases of chronic ulcers or presssure sores.

A blood transfusion is often helpful in improving the patient's general condition and correcting a toxic anaemia.

Clindamycin

Despite its serious side-effects, the first drug to consider is clindamycin. This should be given by mouth in doses of 150–300 mg 6-hourly, or it can be given by intramuscular injection or slow intravenous infusion 600 mg to 2.7 g daily in divided doses. It should not be given in patients with known impairment of hepatic or renal function. The drug should be stopped immediately if the patient develops diarrhoea, for it may cause pseudomembranous colitis. Clindamycin is recommended for staphylococcal bone and joint infections, for it is well concentrated in bone. It is also effective against Gram-positive cocci and many anaerobes.

Flucloxacillin

Flucloxacillin is active in infections due to penicillinase-producing staphylococci, particularly *Staphylococcus aureus*. It is given in doses of 250 mg 6-hourly before food. It may also be given by intramuscular or intravenous injection in the same dosage.

Sodium Fusidate

Another drug which is well concentrated in bone and is active against penicillin-resistant staphylococci is sodium fusidate, which is given by mouth in doses of 500 mg 8-hourly. It may also be given by slow intravenous injection three times a day in doses of 500 mg over 6 hours.

Cephradine

A potentially nephrotoxic drug which is effective against certain Gram-positive and Gram-negative bacteria is cephradine, which may be given orally in doses of 250–500 mg 6-hourly. In severe infections it is better to give it parenterally in doses of 500 mg or 1 g 6-hourly.

These drugs are effective for osteomyelitis following surgery. There is controversy regarding the place of locally applied antibiotics in the treatment of these cases, when the dead tissue is removed.

Aminoglycoside Drugs

When the osteomyelitis follows chronic ulceration or a pressure sore the aminoglycoside drugs are usually used. They have the great disadvantage that they are not absorbed from the gut and have therefore to be given by intramuscular or slow intravenous injection. They are also ototoxic and nephrotoxic and are potentiated by diuretics if the patient is also on these. Gentamicin is the first choice and is given in doses of 2–5 mg/kg body weight in divided doses 8-hourly. Amikacin may be given in doses of 15 mg/kg body weight divided into two doses.

Other antibiotic drugs

Amoxycillin is effective against some Gram-positive and Gram-negative organisms and produces higher plasma and tissue concentrations than ampicillin. It is also absorbed when there is food in the stomach. It is given orally in doses of 250 mg 8-hourly or in the same dose by intramuscular injection.

Metronidazole is very effective against anaerobic bacteria and is given in doses of 400 mg orally 8-hourly. It can also be administered by intravenous infusion or by suppositories *per rectum*.

Isoniazid, Rifampicin and Ethambutol

The treatment of tuberculous osteomyelitis requires a combination of drugs given over a long period. For the first 2 months, at least three drugs are given together (see also Chapter 7).

Isoniazid should be given in doses of 300 mg/day either orally or by intramuscular injection. Its only common side-effect is peripheral neuropathy, but if this does not occur isoniazid should be continued for the whole period of treatment. Rifampicin should be given with the isoniazid. It is given orally before breakfast in doses of 10 mg/kg body weight – a total of usually 450–600 mg. It may cause gastrointestinal symptoms or hepatic complications. Ethambutol is the third drug given in the initial 8 weeks of treatment. It is given orally in doses of 15 mg/kg body weight.

After the initial period only two drugs are used continuously for another 7–16 months. With the isoniazid either rifampicin or ethambutol may be given. In the elderly streptomycin is best avoided due to its tendency to cause ototoxicity and deafness.

Mobilization of Patients

It is a well-accepted principle of geriatric medical practice that there must be a good indication for an elderly patient to be rested, and in the absence of such an indication the patient should be mobilized, albeit gently. In patients with osteomyelitis or pyogenic arthritis rest may well be required at first, particularly after a surgical procedure. A distressed patient in pain requires analgesics to relieve the pain and then regular analgesics to keep him or her pain-free. More analgesic is needed in the first instance to relieve the patient than later to keep the pain away. Pain in the back will be helped with a spinal supporting corset, to allow early ambulation. Rest in bed must be avoided if possible because of the ease with which elderly joints stiffen up and contractures of muscles and tendons occur.

When a patient is on analgesic drugs and is immobilized, there is a likelihood that he will become constipated. This will add to his discomfort, and should be anticipated so that appropriate action can be taken. Bulk, such as vegetables or bran, should be given in his diet, and aperients such as Dorbanex may be prescribed sparingly.

PREVENTION

One of the difficulties of geriatric medicine is that the patient presents for the first time with several disabilities or conditions that are of long-standing. Preventive medicine for the elderly should really be undertaken while the patient is young or middle-aged!

Prompt and effective treatment of infective conditions in the elderly will lessen the risk of haematogenous spread of infection. Where there is a purulent discharge, a swab should be taken and after culture of the organism the appropriate antibiotic should be given. The possibility of tuberculous infection must be borne in mind in elderly men with chronic bronchitis, or in those with a past history of tuberculosis.

The prevention of pressure sores is largely a question of the recognition of those patients who are at risk for developing sores. Immobility, because of diseases like arthritis, will make the patient sit or lie on bony prominences that have only the thinnest overlying subcutaneous tissue and skin. Only by regular relief of this pressure can the thrombosis of the small vessels in the subcutaneous tissue and the consequent death of the skin that they supply be avoided. The first line of treatment is that of good nursing. Only secondarily do devices like alternating pressure mattresses, sorbo or plastic pads, and water beds make a contribution. Mobilization of the patient is of course better than all of this if it is possible. When a pressure sore has occurred, then a determined drive to clean it up, keep it clean and encourage healing is the only way to limit spread of the infection.

Varicose Ulcers

Varicose ulceration can be prevented by adequate early treatment of poor venous return from the legs. In many patients there is a family history of varicose veins, particularly in women. Certain occupations in which there is standing for prolonged periods will provoke varicose veins. Such patients are at risk and should be encouraged to wear supporting stockings at the first sign of trouble. Where the varicose veins are established, surgical treatment may be needed.

Diabetic Patients

Patients with diabetes mellitus are at risk for infections. It follows that good control of their diabetes, either with insulin injections or more usually in elderly patients with hypoglycaemic drugs, will minimize this risk.

Peripheral Vascular Disease

Peripheral obstructive vascular disease is very often associated with heavy cigarette smoking, so advice must be given to stop this. Vasodilator drugs are without value in improving the blood supply, and many other drugs, reputed to improve the nutrition of the tissues, are of unproven value. Where the obstruction is localized vascular surgery in the form of a bypass will reperfuse the arterial bed peripherally, preventing peripheral ischaemia, ulceration and gangrene. Due to great advances in vascular surgery there are now fewer amputations below or above the knee in the elderly for gangrene and ischaemic ulceration.

The prevention of postoperative infection in orthopaedic surgery will depend upon scrupulous attention to aseptic techniques in operating theatres specially designed for bone and joint work. Such sterility is not possible where the operation follows a compound fracture or other severe trauma.

ACKNOWLEDGEMENTS

My thanks are due to J. D. Allison FRCS for Figures 8.1, 8.2 and 8.3, and to Mr R. Maclean for preparing the photographs.

References

1. Waldvogel, F. A., Medoff, G. and Swartz, M. N. (1970). Osteomyelitis. A review of clinical features, therapeutic considerations and unusual aspects. Part one. *N. Engl. J. Med.*, **282,** 198–206
2. Wiley, A. M. and Trueta, J. (1959). The vascular anatomy of the spine and its relationship to pyogenic vertebral osteomyelitis. *J. Bone Jnt. Surg.*, **418,** 796–809
3. Elson , R. A. (1983). *Exchange Arthroplasty for Deep Infection Involving Joint Arthroplasties. Symposium on Joint Arthroplasty.* Belfast, May 1983. International Medicine Supplement 95, p.32
4. Waldvogel, F. A., Medoff, G. and Swartz, M. N. (1970). Osteomyelitis. A review of clinical features, therapeutic considerations and unusual aspects. Part two. *N. Engl. J. Med.*, **282,** 260–6
5. Leading article (1967). Changing character of osteomyelitis. *Br. Med. J.*, **3,** 255–6
6. Bellamy, N., Brooks, P. M. and Austin, T. W. (1983). Septic arthritis. Rheumatology seminar. *Hosp. Update,* 9 November, 1251–68
7. Waldvogel, F. A., Medoff, G. and Swartz, M. N. (1970). Osteomyelitis. A review of clinical features, therapeutic considerations and unusual aspects. Part three. *N. Engl. J. Med.*, **282,** 316–22

9

Central Nervous System Infections in the Elderly

R. J. ANGUS and M. J. DENHAM

BACTERIAL MENINGITIS

Bacterial meningitis, although a relatively rare disease in old age, is even now associated with a high mortality. In the preantibiotic era the mortality rate for all ages exceeded 90% and most survivors were neurologically devastated. Effective antibiotic treatment has reduced the overall mortality rate to about 10–20% but it remains between 50 and 77% for the elderly[1,2].

The graph of mortality from bacterial meningitis related to age for the years 1981–83 shows a bimodal distribution (Figure 9.1). The first peak is, as expected, in infancy but there is also a second peak from 50 to 80 years. Four main factors account for this late peak.

1. The infection may be fulminant and the course so rapid that the patient is referred too late for effective treatment.
2. The diagnosis may be delayed because the illness is attributed to other more common causes.
3. The treatment may be inappropriate.
4. The presence of other pathology may impair the patient's ability to resist the infection.

Improvement in mortality is likely to occur when a high index of suspicion is maintained and when there is better understanding of the principles of treatment.

Factors contributing to increased mortality in pneumococcal meningitis have been analysed[3]. Coexisting illness was found to be the most important

159

factor, but coma, confusion, convulsions, a CSF protein of more than 2.8 g/l and a CSF sugar of less than 0.8 mmol/l were also bad prognostic signs and findings. Indeed, the fatality rate was more than four times as high among patients with associated disease than those with none. In a recent British study[2] 55% of the patients with pneumococcal meningitis had a significant history of conditions associated with impaired resistance to infection such as diabetes mellitus.

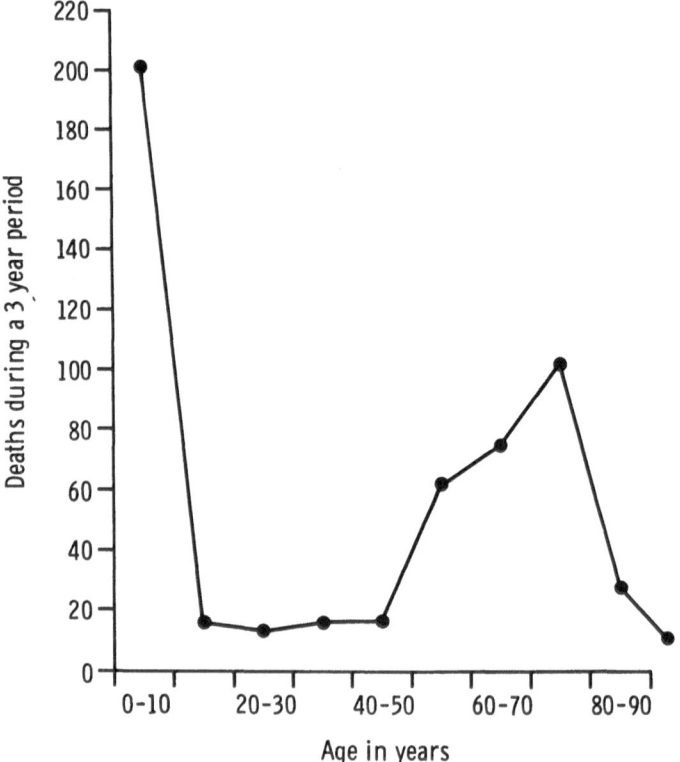

Figure 9.1 Mortality in bacterial meningitis related to age for three years 1981–83. Source: Office of Population Censuses and Surveys (OPCS): *Mortality Statistics*

Incidence

As might be expected the incidence of bacterial meningitis also shows a bimodal distribution which parallels that found in the mortality studies. Data from the Communicable Diseases Surveillance Centre (CDSC) show that of a total number of 1447 cases of meningitis in England and Wales in

1975 only 4.5% were in patients over 65 years[1]. At Northwick Park Hospital, a district general hospital serving a population of 200000 people only eight cases of meningitis in patients over the age of 60 years have been diagnosed by bacteriological or post-mortem evidence in the 13 years between 1970 and 1983. This is probably an underestimate of the true incidence because of the problems not only of diagnosis but also of coding, recording, and retrieval of such data. However, reports show a disturbing increase in the incidence of meningitis in the elderly. Between 1975 and 1978 the number of cases in England and Wales has more than doubled[1]. A similar increase has been noted in the United States[4]. This may represent more vigorous evaluation of confusion, coma and fever.

Predisposing Factors and Bacteriology

Factors predisposing patients to bacterial meningitis are listed in Table 9.1.

Meningitis can follow bacterial seeding of the meninges by contiguous spread from a pericranial focus of infection and direct inoculation of bacteria as a result of head trauma or neurosurgery, but the most common route of infection in the elderly is blood-borne. Fortunately, although bacteraemia is common in elderly patients, few cases result in meningitis.

The site of the primary infection can be useful in indicating the organism causing the meningitis. Pneumonia due to *Streptococcus pneumoniae* is the commonest cause of septicaemia and meningitis in the elderly. *S. pneumoniae* meningitis less frequently follows ear and sinus infections and skull trauma. *Staphylococcus aureus* meningitis can follow neurosurgery, osteomyelitis and cellulitis. Meningitis due to Gram-negative organisms, anaerobes and *Bacteroides* spp., can result from abdominal surgery, urinary tract infections and instrumentation, pressure sores, neurosurgery, osteomyelitis and cellulitis, and those with impaired immunity.

Table 9.1 Factors predisposing to meningitis in the elderly

Local sepsis	Immunoparesis
ear and sinus infection	neoplasia and leukaemia
ear surgery	steroid treatment
head and neck surgery	diabetes mellitus
skull trauma	chronic renal failure
	alcoholism
	splenectomy
	sickle cell disease
Remote sepsis	
pneumonia	
endocarditis	
osteomyelitis	
pyelonephritis	
other septic foci	

Immune-compromised patients have a higher incidence of Gram-negative meningitis and *Listeria monocytogenes* infection. In some cases it may be impossible to demonstrate a predisposing cause. The micro-organisms which cause meningitis in the elderly are listed in Table 9.2. Over half are due to *S. pneumoniae*. *Neisseria meningitidis* and *Listeria monocytogenes* are less common but each occur in about 10% of cases only. The distribution of organisms in Table 9.2 appears constant from year to year in most studies when hospital-acquired infections, particularly in immune-suppressed patients, are included[5]. A British study however, found only one case of *Listeria monocytogenes* in a 10-year retrospective survey[2]. This discrepancy may be due to their selection of patients and exclusion of meningitis associated with cerebral abscess.

Table 9.2 Causative agent of meningitis in patients aged 65 or more in 1978 in England and Wales. (After Newton and Wilczynski[1])

Organism isolated from CSF	Number of cases
Streptococcus pneumoniae	56
Neisseria meningitidis	12
Listeria monocytogenes	11
Escherichia coli	7
Staphylococcus aureus	3
Pseudomonas spp.	3
Klebsiella spp.	3
Streptococcus spp. (others)	2
Haemophilus influenzae	2
Mycobacterium tuberculosis	1
Staphylococcus albus	1
Others	3
	104

Listeria monocytogenes infection typically occurs in the immunosuppressed patient with lymphoproliferative disease and those on steroids. However, listeria meningitis can be lethal in the elderly without underlying disease. Indeed, epidemiological data suggests that age *per se* predisposes to listeria infection perhaps due to age related decrease in cell-mediated immunity. The source of infection in listeria meningitis can often not be identified. About 50% of these patients have associated bacteraemia and in some cases meningitis is associated with pneumonia or otitis media.

Meningitis caused by *Haemophilus influenzae* is extremely rare in the elderly[6] and like *N. meningitidis* it may present in an atypical manner.

Presentation

There is little difficulty in making the diagnosis when there.is a short history of headache and fever with neck stiffness. The history may be as short as 1–3 days in pneumococcal meningitis with rapid deterioration. A rather longer history would suggest infection with one of the less common organisms or *Listeria monocytogenes*. Unfortunately, the elderly patient often presents with malaise and confusion, and many other common conditions may be considered the cause of the illness (Table 9.3). Neck stiffness may be all too easily attributed to cervical spondylosis. However, it should be possible to flex the head at the atlanto-occipital joint in patients with cervical spondylosis and therefore complete rigidity should suggest meningitis or a subarachnoid haemorrhage[7]. The presence of neurological defects and cognitive disorders compound the diagnostic problem since they may be due to a more common pre-existing disease such as cerebrovascular disease, but fluctuation and/or progression of the symptoms should make the clinician suspicious.

Table 9.3 Conditions for which meningitis may be mistaken in the elderly

Cerebral haemorrhage	Hepatic coma
Brain stem haemorrhage	Uraemia
Toxic confusional states	Head injury
Dementia	Subdural haematoma
Hypoglycaemic coma	Cerebral abscess
Hyperosmolar diabetic coma	Cerebral tumour
Intoxication of alcohol or drugs	Post-ictal states

The optic fundi should be assessed for evidence of raised intracranial pressure, choroidal tubercles or haemorrhages associated with bacterial endocarditis. In suspected meningitis slight disc swelling is not a contraindication to lumbar puncture unless accompanied by focal neurological signs or coma, when computerized tomography (CT) should be considered first. The presence of papilloedema makes CT scanning mandatory and lumbar puncture contraindicated.

Although fever is often absent in infective diseases of the elderly, it is almost always present in this situation. Indeed, all eight of the Northwick Park series of cases of meningitis in the elderly were pyrexial on admission. The septicaemic aspects of meningitis may result in the clinical features of pericarditis, arrhythmias, ST depression on e.c.g. and arthralgia, but these may be mistaken for the more commonly occurring ischaemic heart disease or degenerative joint disease.

Rashes, especially those due to antibiotics are all too common in the elderly. Such rashes should be differentiated from the petechial or maculopapular rash of meningococcal infection. A purpuric rash occasionally occurs in pneumococcal infection, and a diffuse pink macular rash can occur on the trunk in listeria infection. Elderly patients with meningococcal meningitis have a better prognosis than those with pneumococcal infection. However, they have a generally worse prognosis than younger patients with the same pathogen and they are more likely to have complications of meningococcal infection, such as the Waterhouse–Friderichsen syndrome, pneumonia, myocarditis and pericarditis.

Investigation of Bacterial Meningitis

The principal investigations are lumbar puncture, blood culture and blood glucose estimation.

Lumbar Puncture

There is no evidence to suggest that the CSF findings differ in any way in the elderly from younger patients either under normal circumstances or in meningitis. The combination of turbidity, pleocytosis, a raised protein level and low glucose level is diagnostic. *Listeria monocytogenes* infection may give a lymphocytic predominance. The Gram-stained smear of centrifuged CSF deposit is vitally important since it may be the only indication of the aetiological organism. *Listeria monocytogenes* is a small Gram-positive rod and has been mistaken for Gram-positive cocci. *Haemophilus influenzae* is sometimes difficult to identify due to Gram-variability and pleomorphism[6].

Blood Cultures

Blood cultures can be a valuable investigation by identifying the causal organism which may fail to grow in the CSF, particularly *Listeria monocytogenes*.

Blood Glucose

Blood glucose should be estimated simultaneously with a CSF glucose since it may detect diabetes precipitated by meningitis. A raised plasma glucose may also cause the CSF glucose to be raised or apparently normal.

Other investigations are of little diagnostic value although countercurrent immunoelectrophoresis sometimes indicates a bacterial antigen in the CSF when other tests are negative.

Treatment of Pyogenic Meningitis by Antibiotics

Meningitis in the elderly is a medical emergency. Urgent, aggressive treatment should be started as soon as the basic investigations have been performed. Since the most likely organisms in the elderly are *S. pneumoniae, N. meningitidis* and *Listeria monocytogenes* high dose intravenous benzylpenicillin 1.2–2.4g (2–4MU) 4-hourly should be given. Postoperative neurosurgical patients or those in whom Gram-negative meningitis is suspected, should be given chloramphenicol 25mg/kg 6-hourly intravenously. Later definitive treatment will be guided by the bacteriological results. Intrathecal antibiotic treatment is unnecessary and potentially dangerous in the common forms of meningitis.

Pneumococcal Meningitis

Most pneumococci are still sensitive to penicillin and high dose intravenous benzyl penicillin should be continued for 7–10 days. Pneumococcal susceptibility to penicillin varies from area to area within Britain and minimal inhibiting concentrations should be determined for all CSF isolates of pneumococci. This is particularly important in patients who do not respond to penicillin treatment. Pneumococci resistant to penicillin and other antibiotics including chloramphenicol have been described[8], but all five patients in that study had received penicillin and/or chloramphenicol for relatively long periods before the resistant pneumococci were cultured. No beta-lactamase was demonstrated in any of the organisms. Other small outbreaks of multiple resistant organisms have been reported, and continued vigilance is required to identify and record such organisms.

Several of the third generation cephalosporins, including cefotaxime, have excellent *in vitro* activity against the pneumococcus, and have good CSF penetration. However, benzylpenicillin remains the drug of choice for pneumococcal meningitis even though its CSF penetration is relatively poor and mortality in the elderly remains high. Patients allergic to penicillin can be treated effectively with chloramphenicol. Combinations of drugs are no longer used routinely.

Meningococcal Meningitis

Sulphonamides are no longer used for initial treatment due to increasing resistance in *N. meningitidis*. The treatment of choice is intravenous benzylpenicillin 1.2–2.4g (2–4MU) 4-hourly. However, a long course of intravenous therapy can sometimes be shortened by using oral sulphadiazine, sulphadimidine or sulphafurazole if the organism is sensitive.

Listeria monocytogenes Meningitis

Although the antibiotic sensitivity of strains of *Listeria monocytogenes* varies, treatment with either penicillin or ampicillin is effective. Penicillin can therefore be given before the bacteriological results are available.

Gram-negative Meningitis

Chloramphenicol is the treatment of choice for *H. influenzae* meningitis, since about 10% of *H. influenzae* isolates produce beta-lactamase which inactivates ampicillin. If bacteriological testing shows that the organism is fully sensitive to ampicillin then this drug can be substituted for chloramphenicol.

Gram-negative meningitis due to organisms other than *H. influenzae* presents a difficult antibiotic choice. Ampicillin and chloramphenicol were the mainstays of treatment but since approximately 30% of *Escherichia coli* causing adult meningitis are ampicillin-resistant, this treatment was often combined with gentamicin. The CSF penetration of aminoglycosides does not allow CSF concentrations adequate to kill the bacteria if gentamicin is given systemically. Even lumbar intrathecal administration is unreliable in achieving effective levels. The use of chloramphenicol is controversial because it has bacteriostatic rather than bacteriocidal activity and it can cause bone marrow aplasia. The newer cephalosporins show promise in the treatment of this clinical problem. Latamoxef (Moxalactam) and cefotaxime are two that have been studied in connection with Gram-negative bacillary meningitis[9,10]. Both drugs have excellent activity against many Gram-negative organisms and penetrate the CSF in bacteriocidal concentrations when given systemically. The efficacy of Moxalactam in meningitis is essentially limited to *H. influenzae, E. coli,* klebsiella, and some proteus infections. It is ineffective against pseudomonas. Cefotaxime has a similar spectrum of activity, but also offers activity against streptococci other than group D streptococci. Specific sensitivity testing of the *E. coli,* klebsiella, and proteus species against these drugs should always be performed. Sensitivity of the organisms cannot be assumed, particularly in case of nosocomial Gram-negative bacillary meningitis.

Treatment of Pyogenic Meningitis – other Measures

Steroids have limited value since cerebral oedema secondary to infection is not reduced[11] and indeed they may also render the blood–brain barrier less permeable to antimicrobial agents.

Fits should be controlled with short-term anticonvulsants such as phenytoin. Phenobarbitone should be avoided because it may blur evaluation of mental state.

Repeating lumbar puncture routinely to assess progress is not recommended since it may be harmful in promoting further symptoms and unnecessary changes in treatment[9]. It should only be repeated if persistent infection is suspected.

Pneumococcal vaccines have been used to improve mortality in patients over 50 years of age with recurrent respiratory problems, and those with underlying disease such as diabetes, chronic cardiac failure or renal insufficiency. However, the incidence of different pneumococcal serotypes varies with time, geographical area, the age of the patient and the disease process. In general the vaccine is less effective and long-lasting in the elderly and antibody response to vaccination should be established when possible. Failure of vaccination to prevent vaccine-type infection and meningitis has been reported even though antibody response was documented[12].

CEREBRAL ABSCESS

The incidence of cerebral abscess is also bimodally distributed. One peak occurs in the first two decades and the second in the two decades between 50 and 70[13]. In a group of 24 patients whose abscesses were diagnosed only at post-mortem examination, one-third were over 60 years. The ratio of men to women was 2:1.

Early diagnosis and treatment is extremely important because antibiotic response is more effective before capsule formation occurs round the abscess thus reducing the need for neurosurgery.

Predisposing Factors

Cerebral abscesses arise from blood-borne infection or local spread from infections arising from either outside the body, as in penetrating injuries or neurosurgery, or from inside such as teeth or paranasal sinus infections. However, in 25% of cases the site of the original infection remains unknown, perhaps because of widespread antibiotic use which eliminates the primary infection but not the cerebral abscess. Nearly a quarter of fatal cases of cerebral abscess have bacterial endocarditis[13]. In some patients the abscess appears to progress even though appropriate antibiotic treatment is given.

Diagnosis

The predominant presenting features are those of an expanding intracerebral lesion with headache and focal signs rather than an infectious process[13]. While there are no special features of cerebral abscesses in the elderly, the symptoms and signs may once again be attributed to other more common conditions. Other pre-existing diseases serve only to complicate the situation. Fever is frequently absent, and the peripheral leukocyte count is frequently lower than 10 000 per mm³. Many patients present with a major central nervous system deficit including hemiparesis, visual field defect, cerebellar syndrome or fits. The signs develop subacutely over 1 or 2 weeks, but still may be mistaken for a cerebrovascular incident, due to rapid development of oedema surrounding the abscess. The diagnostic clue of neck stiffness is present in about 50% of cases, due either to raised intracranial pressure or associated meningitis. Experience with other intracranial space occupying lesions indicates that papilloedema is not always present in the elderly when it might be expected due to the compensatory presence of cerebral atrophy. Absence of papilloedema, therefore, does not rule out cerebral abscess.

Lumbar Puncture

Lumbar puncture should be avoided in patients with the features of cerebral abscess because of the risk of tentorial herniation. However, when CSF is examined it may be normal, show a leukocytosis or frank meningitis, but culture is rarely rewarding. In some cases the abscess may rupture into the ventricular system resulting in meningitis. This carries a poor prognosis.

Computerized Tomography

This is helpful in diagnosis and assessing response to treatment. A routine scan shows only an area of hypoattenuation and the mass effect of the abscess. Contrast enhancement shows a ring around the abscess due to release of contrast into areas of increased vascular permeability surrounding the focus[14]. Nuclear magnetic resonance scanning may prove a more sensitive diagnostic technique. Instillation of radio-opaque material into the abscess cavity is obsolete because it interferes with subsequent CT scanning.

Management

Antibiotics and neurosurgery form the basis of management of cerebral abscess although the timing of neurosurgery is debatable.

Antibiotic Treatment

The microbiology of intracranial abscesses is complex with both facultative and obligate anaerobes and carbon dioxide-dependent bacteria. Multiple organisms are recovered from up to 60% of cases[13]. Consequently combination antibiotic therapy will be needed until the causal organism or organisms have been identified.

Since the commonest organisms are streptococci, most of which are penicillin-sensitive, intravenous benzyl penicillin 1.2–2.4 g (2–4 MU) should be given 4-hourly. This is combined with systemic metronidazole to cover obligate anaerobes, especially anaerobic streptococci and bacteroides. This antimicrobial agent is not susceptible to beta-lactamase and penetrates the CSF and brain tissue well. Chloramphenicol is added to this regime because of its superior penetration of the blood–brain barrier and to cover *Haemophilus* species which are often isolated alone or as part of mixed flora, particularly in cases of chronic sinusitis. The Enterobacteriaceae, especially *E. coli* and *Proteus* species, are often found in mixed cultures of post-traumatic or post-neurosurgical abscesses, or of abscesses associated with chronic otitis. In these cases gentamicin should be added or one of the newer cephalosporin-related compounds. If trauma or osteomyelitis is thought to be the cause of the abscess the treatment should include an antistaphylococcal drug, for example an isoxazolyl penicillin, or vancomycin in penicillin allergy. Treatment should continue for at least 6 weeks.

Neurosurgery

Techniques and attitudes vary. Some neurosurgeons recommend primary excision of the abscess followed by chemotherapy[14]. Others favour simple aspiration and chemotherapy, except in cerebellar abscesses[15]. However, once abscess formation has occurred, surgical intervention is the only definitive method for eradicating infection inaccessible to antibiotics, and for preventing the pressure-related complications of brain abscess.

Anticonvulsants

Anticonvulsants are prescribed routinely because the risk of fits is high not only during the illness, but also as a later complication. They should be continued for at least 5 years.

Steroids

Dexamethasone may be used to control cerebral oedema, but the use of steroids remains controversial because of their adverse effect on the diffusion of antibiotics to the site of infection.

Prognosis

Untreated cerebral abscess results in 100% mortality. The mortality of treated abscesses varies from 30 to 50% depending on the age and general condition of the patient, pre-existing diseases, the virulence of the organism and the risks of neurosurgery. Of the survivors, 50% have seizures, 50% have neurological deficits and 10% are totally incapacitated.

TUBERCULOUS MENINGITIS

Formerly a complication of primary infection in infancy and childhood, tuberculous meningitis (TBM) is now seen in adults as a result of reactivated disease in the central nervous system. It is less often a part of miliary disease and more commonly a reactivation and rupture of a caseous focus or tubercle in the meninges, cerebral or spinal tissue. The subsequent development depends on the inflammatory reaction and the ischaemia and infarction resulting from arteritis.

Incidence and Mortality

The overall incidence of tuberculous meningitis in England and Wales is 30 cases per year, but less than 10% of these are elderly. In a study of TBM in Glasgow, Kennedy[16] found that five out of 52 cases were over 50 years old and three of these died. The high mortality was due to the usual factors of delay in diagnosis and presence of underlying disease[17].

Tuberculous meningitis is particularly common in Asians and language difficulties may add to the diagnostic problem. However, it also occurs in Caucasians especially where there is a history of tuberculous contact[18]. Kennedy[16] found that over half of the cases had close contact with tuberculosis. The contacts in 21% of these were receiving or had recently received treatment, and 25% were regarded as cured.

Clinical Features

The clinical presentation is of a subacute meningitis with symptoms of tuberculous toxaemia. Initially the symptoms are non-specific with general malaise, low grade fever, anorexia, vague intermittent headaches and muscle pains. The elderly have symptoms of a toxic confusional state with fluctuating confusion, personality change and drowsiness. After a few weeks more definite neurological features develop including persistent headache, neck stiffness, oculomotor palsies, hemiparesis and sometimes tremor and involuntary movements. Choroidal tubercles are only seen as part of miliary diseases.

Progressive coma, multiple cranial nerve palsies and hemiplegia are features associated with poor prognosis.

Lumbar Puncture

Absolute confirmation of the diagnosis of tuberculous meningitis depends on the identification of *Mycobacterium tuberculosis* in the CSF, although this is only achieved in uder 40% of initial specimens[17]. The cell count typically rises to 400/mm^3, mainly lymphocytes, and the protein concentration rises from 0.8 to 4.0 g/l. The glucose level falls, sometimes to zero. However, proven cases of TBM with tubercle bacilli in the CSF have been associated with normal CSF findings in patients who are severely ill, on steroids or in those in whom immunological function is impaired. However, 48 hours later the CSF has shown the usual abnormalities. Consequently, when clinical suspicion is high, lumbar puncture should be repeated 24 hours after a normal result. Encouraging results from a new agglutination test for plasma membrane antigen in CSF to *M. tuberculosis* in childhood TBM[19] require further evaluation in adults.

Other Investigations

A chest X-ray may provide important information. Kennedy[16] found miliary changes in about 40% of cases. Other tests, such the white cell count in the peripheral blood, can be of little value, and the ESR may be entirely normal in elderly patients. The tuberculin reaction may be negative. A history of past immunization with BCG vaccine may be misleading and does not preclude the diagnosis of tuberculous meningitis.

Treatment

Chemotherapy

Four antituberculous drugs should be given initially until sensitivities are available. Only isonicotinic acid hydrazide (INAH), ethionamide and pyrazinamide penetrate non-inflamed meninges effectively. Rifampicin, ethambutol and systemically administered streptomycin only penetrate if the meninges are inflamed in the first 4–6 weeks of the illness. Streptomycin 1 g/day intramuscularly is given with INAH 300–600 mg/day, rifampicin 600 mg/day and pyrazinamide 40 mg/kg/day. The latter three drugs should be given orally or by nasogastric tube in comatose patients. Intrathecal use of streptomycin is nowadays usually omitted. Chemotherapy is usually continued for 18–24 months, since there is no evidence that shorter courses are both safe and effective.

If a positive bacteriological diagnosis of TBM cannot be made and the possibility of pyogenic meningitis remains, a severely ill patient should be treated with penicillin in addition to the full antituberculous regime until the diagnosis is clarified.

The problem of drug compliance in the elderly is well known and close supervision is required to prevent development of resistant organisms. Toxic effects are also more common in the elderly, particularly liver toxicity with rifampicin and INAH[16]. Renal failure may result in higher than expected levels of ethambutol, thus potentiating the development of optic neuritis; ototoxicity of streptomycin is also more likely with renal insufficiency. INAH interferes with the metabolism of other drugs such as phenytoin which may be needed to control fits. Serum levels of phenytoin should be monitored regularly to prevent toxicity which may result in somnolence, ataxia, vestibulo-ocular disturbances and behavioural changes.

Steroids

The place of steroids in treating TBM is debatable[20]. No properly controlled trial of their use exists. Dexamethasone is probably justified in very ill patients, those with cerebral oedema, adrenal failure or severe drug reactions, and in those suspected of developing hydrocephalus or spinal block. However, steroids complicate management by suppressing the characteristic response to treatment, by producing a sense of wellbeing and by increasing the risk of secondary infection and electrolyte disturbance. Steroids also restore the blood–brain barrier, thus diminishing drug penetration.

Neurosurgery

This contributes to a favourable outcome in patients who have pronounced cerebral oedema[17].

Intracranial Tuberculoma

Tuberculomas are usually single and behave as space-occupying lesions. A minority develop in the course of TBM even during antituberculous treatment[21]. A high proportion of patients are Asian[22]. Diagnosis may be difficult in the absence of fever and malaise, but a past history of tuberculosis, contact with it or evidence of tuberculosis outside the CNS is helpful. However, nearly 70% of cases have a normal chest X-ray[22]. The clinical course of tuberculomas has no features distinguishing them from other space-occupying lesions of the brain. Comparison of tuberculomas with gliomas revealed no significantly different features[23].

Computerized tomography has been a major advance in the diagnosis and management of intracranial tuberculoma. Calcification is the only feature which distinguishes a tuberculoma from an abscess, but this does not develop until the lesion is healing. Tuberculomas appear as low attenuation or isodense lesions of variable size on CT scan[22]. Enhancement is predominantly uniform or irregular but it can occasionally be ring-shaped. There is variable surrounding oedema and features of space occupation.

Treatment

Treatment is similar to that of tuberculous meningitis. A trial of antituberculous therapy should be given without biopsy confirmation of the diagnosis in those patients where there is very high clinical suspicion. Improvement in clinical and CT features can be monitored and avoids the need for surgery which is then reserved for patients who do not respond to medical treatment.

References

1. Newton, J. E. and Wilczynski, P. J. G. (1979). Meningitis in the elderly. *Lancet 2*, 157
2. Davey, P. G., Cruikshank, J. K., McManus, I. C., Mahood, B., Snow, M. H. and Geddes, A. M. (1982). Bacterial meningitis – ten years experience. *J. Hyg. Camb.*, **88**, 383
3. Weiss, W., Figueroa, W. Shapiro, W. H. and Flippin, H. F. (1967). Prognostic factors in pneumococcal meningitis. *Arch. Intern. Med.*, **120**, 517
4. Fraser, D. W., Henke, C. E. and Feldman, R. A. (1973). Changing patterns of bacterial meningitis in Olmstead County, Minnesota 1935–1970. *J. Infect. Dis.*, **128**, 300
5. Massanari, R. M. (1977). Purulent meningitis in the elderly: when to suspect an unusual pathogen. *Geriatrics*, **32**, 55
6. Eykyn, S. J., Thomas, R. D. and Phillips, I. (1974). *Haemophilus influenzae* meningitis in adults. *Br. Med. J.*, **2**, 463
7. Coakley, D. (1981). *Acute Geriatric Medicine.* (London: Croom Helm)
8. Appelbaum, P. C., Scragg, J. N., Bowen, A. J., Bhanijee, A., Hallett, A. F. and Cooper, R. C. (1977). *Streptococcus pneumoniae* resistant to penicillin and chloramphenicol. *Lancet*, **2**, 995
9. Lambert, M. P. (1983). Treatment of bacterial meningitis. *Br. Med. J.*, **286**, 741
10. Beam, T. R. (1984). Cephalosporins in adult meningitis. *Bull. NY Acad. Med.*, **60**, 380
11. Editorial (1982). Steroids in bacterial meningitis – helpful or harmful. *Lancet*, **1**, 1164
12. Patel, K. M. (1981). Pneumococcal meningitis – occurrence after vaccination in an elderly patient. *Aust. NW J. Med.*, **11**, 564

13. Brewer, N. S., MacCarty, C. S. and Wellman, W. E., (1975). Brain abscess: a review of recent experience. *Ann. Intern. Med.*, **82,** 571
14. Garvey, G. (1983). Current concepts of bacterial infections of the central nervous system. *J. Neurosurg.*, **59,** 735
15. Editorial (1978). Chemotherapy of brain abscess. *Lancet*, **2,** 1081
16. Kennedy, D. H. and Fallon, R. J., (1979). Tuberculous meningitis. *J. Am. Med. Assoc.*, **241,** 264
17. Fallon, R. J. and Kennedy, D. H., (1981). Treatment and prognosis in tuberculous meningitis. *J. Infect.*, **3,** Suppl. **1,** 39
18. Traub, M., Colchester, A. C. F., Kingsley, D. P. E. and Swash, M. (1984). Tuberculosis of the central nervous system. *Q. J. Med.*, **209,** 81
19. Krambovitis, E., Lock, P. E., McIllmurray, M. B., Hendrickse, W. and Holzel, H., (1984). Rapid diagnosis of tuberculous meningitis by latex particle agglutination. *Lancet*, **2,** 1229
20. Gordon, A. and Parsons, M. (1972). The place of corticosteroids in the management of tuberculous meningitis. *Br. J. Hosp. Med.*, **7,** 651
21. Lees, A. J. MacLeod, A. F. and Marshall, J. (1980). Cerebral tuberculomas developing during treatment of tuberculous meningitis. *Lancet*, **1,** 1208
22. Loizou, L. A. and Anderson, M. (1982). Intracranial tuberculomas: correlation of computerised tomography with clinico-pathological findings. *Q. J. Med.*, **201,** 104
23. Dastur, H. M. and Desai, A. D. (1965). A comparative study of brain tuberculomas and gliomas based upon 107 case records of each. *Brain*, **88,** 375

10

Herpes Simplex and Varicella Zoster Virus Infection in the Elderly

T. E. A. PETO and B. E. JUEL-JENSEN

Herpes viruses are widespread throughout the animal kingdom. Characteristically, one or more herpes viruses live in harmless symbiosis with their host. For instance, the oyster and the cobra have their own herpes viruses. However, if a herpes virus by accident gets into the 'wrong' host it may cause much damage. Simian herpes virus, whose host is certain old-world monkeys, may cause lethal encephalomyelitis in man, when its normal host is rarely ill.

Man is host to four herpes viruses: varicella zoster and its close cousin herpes simplex virus (HSV), both of which become latent in nerve cells. Cytomegalovirus and Epstein–Barr viruses rarely give rise to disease in the elderly unless they become immunosuppressed from whatever cause. Varicella zoster virus is the most important herpes virus in the elderly because of the often devastating pain shingles causes in those over 60. All are characterized by a primary attack in the non-immune host. The virus becomes latent and later may become reactivated; this happens commonly in herpes simplex, more rarely in varicella zoster and hardly ever in cytomegalovirus and Epstein–Barr virus infection.

VARICELLA ZOSTER

Primary Infection

Chickenpox is rare in the elderly because most adults in the western world are immune; 90% of Oxford clinical students have detectable serum anti-

175

body to varicella zoster and by the age of 65 this is probably nearer 100%. Varicella zoster virus, however, is less prevalent in tropical and semitropical countries and older inhabitants from these regions may well get chickenpox. This pattern is becoming more common in the temperate regions as the incidence of chickenpox in the upper socioeconomic groups decreases. Chickenpox is highly infectious and within families there is at least a 75% 'hit' rate in non-immune contacts. Patients remain infectious until all the vesicles have dried, although they are most infectious in the early part of the illness.

Clinical Features

When chickenpox does occur, it is likely to be more severe in adults than in children. It is spread by air droplets or contact with the vesicles and has a median incubation period of 14 days. The prodromal illness, the time of maximal viral replication, consists of fever, headache, malaise and myalgia and lasts for 2–3 days; a longer and more severe prodrome heralds a more severe disease. The rash, which is intensely itchy, typically is centripetal. There are lesions on the trunk, both over bony prominences and in parts that are not exposed to pressure. The rash usually starts on the back and progresses to the trunk, arms and legs and finally the face. Each spot goes through a cycle (macule, papule, vesicle and finally crust formation) which takes about 8–24 hours. Normally several fresh crops of spots appear during the illness. In uncomplicated cases the illness should resolve over about a week.

In older patients cases are easily diagnosed clinically. There is often a known contact with chickenpox or shingles. In difficult cases, electron microscopy of vesicular fluid, preferably taken in a capillary tube, will demonstrate particles typical of the herpes group, and growth in tissue culture after 3–4 days will allow type specification. A four-fold or greater rise in titres to varicella zoster virus antibody in paired sera is also diagnostic. Since the extinction of smallpox there is no main diagnostic difficulty although it should be remembered that the other poxviruses, such as monkeypox and Tanapox, are still present in remote areas of Central and East Africa. Mild cases may be confused with transient vesicular rashes of the enteroviruses, in particular hand, foot and mouth disease, and, very rarely, cytomegalovirus. More confluent rashes may be due to drug eruptions. If there is *any* doubt about whether a patient might have a poxvirus, he must at 'once be sent to an infectious diseases unit for isolation.

Complications

The overall mortality of chickenpox is one in 30 000 but this is higher in adults and is likely to be even higher in the elderly, although no exact figures are available. In severe cases, the prodrome can be like smallpox with severe pain in both back and loin; a transient pink rash occurring 2–4 days before the main eruption is a poor prognostic sign.

Pneumonitis

Pneumonitis presents with a cough, chest pain, breathlessness or haemoptysis 2–3 days after the onset of the rash. In fulminating cases death ensues within 24–48 hours. In most cases, the course is less severe and in some the pneumonitis can only be detected radiologically. The changes of diffuse patchy infiltration occasionally persist for months or years and are benign. The multiple calcification seen on subsequent chest X-rays, said to be characteristic of chickenpox, are unusual.

Encephalitis

Varicella encephalitis is rare. It occurs within a week of the appearance of the rash, presenting with headache, vomiting, convulsions, ataxia and signs of raised intracranial pressure. Cranial nerve palsies may develop. The cerebrospinal fluid shows lymphocytosis, raised protein and usually normal 'sugar', although a lowered 'sugar' has been reported. In severe cases there is a rapid progression to coma and death but it should be realized that complete recovery from coma is always possible. Lumbar puncture should never be undertaken unless cerebral oedema has been excluded by computerized tomography (CT scan).

Other Complications

Secondary infection of the spots is common but not very serious. Rarely thrombocytopenia occurs causing 'haemorrhagic chickenpox'. A very rare complication is purpura fulminans when immune complexes damage the small vessel walls, there is profound thrombocytopenia and often extensive tissue loss. Hepatitis with clinical jaundice occurs occasionally in older patients.

Immunosuppressed Patients

Chickenpox in patients who are already immunosuppressed is much more severe. Cell-mediated immunity as well as humoral immunity is important in the control of the infection. Patients with lymphoproliferative disease (lymphoma, lymphoblastic leukaemia, Hodgkin's disease, multiple myeloma and other reticuloses) or who are treated with steroids, cytotoxic or other immunosuppressive agents are at high risk. The disease often affects the whole body and can damage the heart, liver, joints, spleen, bladder, ureters, kidney or central nervous system.

Management

Simple management is often all that is required with antipyretics, antihistamines for itch and calamine lotion for the rash. Secondary infection should be treated with antibiotics. If the chickenpox is severe, or there are visceral complications, parenteral antiviral chemotherapy should be given immediately. High dose intravenous acyclovir (10 mg/kg 8-hourly) infused over not less than 1 hour is given for 5 days. Lower doses are given in renal failure. Patients with pneumonitis may require ventilating. Hyperimmune varicella zoster virus globulin is of doubtful value except, possibly, in cases where there is pre-existing hypogammaglobulinaemia with a real doubt as to whether the patient can raise antibodies. Patients requiring admission to hospital should ideally be admitted to an infectious diseases unit, or in any case be nursed in isolation away from immunocompromised patients and pregnant mothers, who are at special risk. If such people are exposed, they can be protected by prophylactic administration of hyperimmune varicella zoster virus globulin within 48 hours of contact. Hyperimmune varicella zoster virus globulin is not recommended for normal healthy people.

SHINGLES (ZOSTER)

Chickenpox is typically an illness of children. Shingles, by contrast, is typically an illness of the elderly. After the primary infection the virus is thought to remain latent in the sensory and motor ganglia. After a variable period of time reactivation occurs, normally from one ganglion, giving rise to shingles. The exact trigger is not known but it is thought to be due to a depression of cell-mediated immunity to varicella zoster virus. There is no evidence that occult malignancy ever presents as shingles[1]. The humoral immunity probably prevents haematogenous spread; in the elderly antibodies are often absent during the first few days of the illness and there may be a generalized rash. In a few cases specific triggers such as trauma, local radiotherapy and ultraviolet light can be identified. Chickenpox can be caught from zoster vesicles; shingles patients are less infectious than those with chickenpox and there is a 'hit' rate of about 15% within families.

Incidence

The incidence of shingles in otherwise healthy people is age related, rising from four per 1000 per year at 55 years to ten per 1000 per year at 90 years of age, with no difference between the sexes. It is likely that at least a quarter of people over 65 will suffer from shingles at some time, and it has been estimated that if you have had chickenpox in childhood and live to be 100 you will certainly get shingles. It is unusual for healthy people to get a second attack of shingles: only about 4% of patients, usually the very old, give a history of a previous attack[2,3]. Few people have any recollection of having had chickenpox in the past.

Presentation

Typically, there is a prodromal paraesthesia, with symptoms of burning, pricking or tenderness to touch over a single dermatome. Fresh vesicles are seen over a few days. Pain is common and can be very severe. It usually starts a few days before the eruption, but may begin as long as 3 weeks before. It persists for 1–2 weeks; unfortunately it can sometimes persist for much longer ('postherpetic neuralgia'; see below). After a few days there is a skin eruption, initially of macules (sometimes confluent), rapidly progressing to vesicles and then crusting after several more days. Fresh vesicles erupt over the first few days of the illness. The vesicles, especially if neglected, are often superinfected with *Staphyloccus aureus* with golden yellow encrustations. Shingles is usually accompanied by a systemic illness consisting of mild fever (up to 38° C) and malaise; there is a mild thrombocytopenia but there is no change in the peripheral white blood cell count or erythrocyte sedimentation rate (ESR). In about 30% of cases, a few vesicles are seen outside the dermatome (satellite lesions) and are not a sign of generalized dissemination. In some cases no rash ever appears (*'zoster sine herpete'*), and the only symptom of disease may be pain or dermatomal hyperaesthesia. This can be confused with cord lesions and even myocardial pain. It cannot be overemphasized that shingles, primarily, is a disease of the *nerve,* both sensory and motor (see below), and, though fascinating for the patient and doctor, the vesicles are of very minor importance.

Diagnosis

Apart from *zoster sine herpete,* the clinical diagnosis is usually easy. The only important condition not to be confused with shingles is zosteriform herpes simplex. Often there is a history of recurrent attacks in the same dermatome and sometimes the lesions are bilateral; both features are rare in shingles.

The diagnosis of shingles, as in chickenpox, can be confirmed by growing the varicella zoster virus from vesicle fluid or by demonstrating it by electron microscopy. A four-fold or greater rise in antibody in acute and convalescent sera is diagnostic.

Complications

Motor and Autonomic Zoster

Occasionally varicella zoster virus affects only a motor nerve. Lower motor neurone facial palsy is the commonest, and is usually associated with sensory zoster of branches of C2 or the trigeminal nerve, and usually takes several weeks to resolve if it resolves at all. Segmental cutaneous zoster can be associated with motor weakness of the corresponding or neighbouring segment. Sacral shingles can present before the onset of the rash, with haemorrhagic cystitis and acute retention of urine. Cystitis presents with dysuria, frequency and haematuria and usually runs a relatively short and benign course; characteristic vesicles may be visualized on cystoscopy. Acute retention presents with a history of several days of difficulty in micturition followed a few days later with a typical rash in the sacral dermatomes; cystoscopy is usually normal, though severe haemorrhagic cystitis is seen occasionally with typical vesicles. Acute retention of urine can sometimes be accompanied by severe constipation due to hypomobility of the rectum. Zoster retention can run a protracted course; this may be due to a granulomatous prostatitis caused by infiltration of varicella zoster virus and may require prostatectomy. Lumbar shingles may lead to hypomobility of the colon. The so called 'Ramsay–Hunt syndrome', a postulated zoster of sensory fetal fibres of the facial nerve and geniculate ganglion, does not exist and should be relegated to the area of herpetiform romance.

Ophthalmic Zoster

When shingles affects the first division of the trigeminal nerve, the eye may be involved, but usually only when the nasociliary branch of the ophthalmic nerve is involved. Oedema of the eyelids, often spreading to the other side, is worrying for the patient but is only due to the tightness of the fascial plane in the forehead which forces the oedema fluid into the loose tissues of the orbit. In a recent series of 61 cases of ocular zoster[4] where no specific antiviral treatment was given, 47 had keratitis, 37 had uveitis leading to 11 instances of secondary glaucoma and seven of cataract. Only three developed extra-ocular palsies but, alarmingly, two developed a contralateral hemiplegia due to granulomatous angiitis, and another three developed cerebral arteritis.

These changes were associated with the presence of varicella zoster virus found in the artery. About 25% of the patients suffered some visual impairment and some 12% of the patients eventually required tarsorrhaphy. Complete loss of vision from shingles is rare.

Postherpetic Neuralgia

Postherpetic neuralgia is the most dreaded of the complications of shingles and occurs in about 10% of all untreated patients, but in about 30–40% of patients over 65. Of these, some 45% have pain for less than 8 weeks and 22% have pain for more than a year. The incidence of pain is lowest with lumbar zoster and is highest in ophthalmic zoster.

Generalized Zoster

Because most elderly patients have no detectable varicella zoster virus antibodies during the first few days of the disease, a few blood-borne skin lesions are common. Occasionally the haematogenous spread may be massive but, provided the patient is not immunosuppressed, the rash is harmless and, once antibodies appear, new lesions cease. The rash resembles chickenpox and the disease only becomes severe if there is visceral involvement. Patients on anticoagulants may bleed into the lesions, or they may also bleed into nervous tissue affected by the virus, for example the spinal cord.

Zoster Encephalitis

Zoster encephalitis is unusual but occurs more often in immunosuppressed patients[5]. Encephalitis occurs normally about 1 week after the onset of the rash but it can occur as early as 4 weeks before and as late as 8 weeks after the onset of the rash. The encephalitis, sometimes accompanied by cutaneous dissemination, is characterized by delirium or hallucinations with signs of meningeal irritation. There is a high incidence of cerebellar ataxia and about a third of patients have cranial or extracranial nerve palsies. The encephalitis usually resolves after 2–3 weeks, though ataxia persists for a few weeks longer. The mortality rate is about 20% but if the patients recover they rarely suffer any long-term sequelae.

The diagnosis of zoster encephalitis is often made by exclusion of other causes because it is a difficult diagnosis to confirm. Examination of the cerebrospinal fluid is not very helpful because a lymphocytosis occurs in about 50% of patients with uncomplicated zoster; recovery of the virus is unusual and has also been reported in patients with uncomplicated zoster.

The diagnosis can be important when encephalopathy occurs in patients who have already received a course of antiviral treatment; in such cases the encephalopathy may be due to the side-effects from the treatment. If encephalitis is suspected no lumbar puncture should be performed until cerebral oedema has been excluded by CT scan. The only certain way of diagnosing varicella zoster virus encephalitis is by brain biopsy, a less traumatic procedure than imagined by many; varicella zoster virus can be demonstrated quickly in brain tissue by immunofluorescence.

Immunocompromised Patients

Patients with lymphoproliferative diseases or acquired immune deficiency, or those treated with steroids, cytotoxic drugs or other immunosupressant agents, have decreased cell-mediated immunity and are at increased risk from zoster[6]. All complications seem to be more prevalent. In one series of 107 patients[7], dissemination occurred in 15% of cases about 4–11 days after the onset of the local lesions, with a mortality of 6% once dissemination had occurred. The overall mortality in these patients varies from 0 to 5% in different series which have looked at all age groups. It would seem likely that the elderly would again be at increased risk. Non-fatal visceral complications are more common than in otherwise healthy patients. The main complication is in the central nervous system, occurring in more than 5% of immunosuppressed patients, and presenting with encephalitis, meningitis, myelitis or peripheral neuropathies.

Management

Patients should be nursed away from immunosuppressed patients and pregnant women because of the risk of chickenpox. The management of shingles is controversial and rapidly changing because of the development of new and expensive antiviral drugs. Uncomplicated shingles is often mild and simple nursing and analgesia may be all that is required. The lesions are kept dry and soothed with calamine. Unfortunately, it is not possible to predict which patients will suffer from postherpetic neuralgia. It is our practice, therefore, to apply topical idoxuridine (35%) in dimethylsulphoxide (DMSO) daily for 5 days occlusively with lint. Treatment reduces the duration and severity of pain but is only effective if it is started within a day of onset of fresh vesicles or at least within 5 days of onset of the rash[8]. The DMSO, itself bactericidal, also has the added advantage of keeping the area sterile. DMSO releases histamine in the skin which causes some reddening and irritation; 5% of patients, however, get histamine vesicles which can be treated with antihistamines; they disappear when DMSO is stopped. In cases of DMSO intolerance, it may be necessary to abandon treatment and substitute systemic medication. Infected zoster is treated with topical antiseptics, but in severe cases topical Fucidin is given perhaps occasionally with the addition of oral flucloxacillin. The lesions are kept dry and scratching discouraged as it can cause scarring.

Complicated shingles (motor, autonomic, sacral, ophthalmic or disseminated) cannot be treated topically and should have systemic antiviral treatment. Immunosuppressed patients should be routinely treated systemically to avoid systemic complications. At the present time there is no good oral agent available, and for elderly patients high dose acyclovir is the drug of choice (10 mg/kg 8-hourly for 5 days; infusions are given over at least 1 hour to avoid crystalluria, and lower doses are given when the creatinine clearance falls below 50 ml/min[9-11]. Vidarabine (ARA-A) is perhaps more active against the virus but is less well tolerated in the elderly, for it may produce a tiresome Parkinsonian tremor. Acyclovir, and to a greater extent, vidarabine are poorly soluble in water and must be given in large volumes of fluid. Because patients with heart disease may be pushed into heart failure, loop diuretics are given prophylactically. It should not be forgotten that cytarabine (ARA-C), which is one of the few soluble antiherpetic drugs, is as effective as idoxuridine against varicella zoster virus. It can be given safely at a dose of 3 mg/kg/day, but as it causes nausea it should be reserved for rare special cases. Bromovinyl deoxyuridine may be a superior drug and should be considered in life-threatening infection. Its potential deserves further exploration[12].

One problem with antiviral treatment is that it is expensive and difficult to administer; shingles unfortunately is very common. Some clinicians feel that the disease, which is rarely fatal, does not warrant such difficult treatment. Shingles, however, is a highly unpleasant disease and causes a great deal of distress and fear in the elderly. We believe that good nursing as well as agressive antiviral treatment can reduce a lot of 'silent suffering' in the community. There is, however, an urgent need for better, simpler, and cheaper antiviral drugs.

All patients with ocular zoster should be examined ophthalmologically with the aid of a slit lamp and the complications treated appropriately with topical steroids, antibiotics and mydriatics. It is our policy to treat all such cases with specific parenteral antiviral treatment to reduce the incidence and severity of these complications. Furthermore we believe that the use of topical steroids alone, early in the course of the disease when the virus is still replicating, will increase the severity of the disease, and we always use topical antiviral cream or drops (idoxuridine or vidarabine).

Zoster encephalitis complicated by cerebral oedema or cranial nerve palsies should be treated by agents that lower intracranial pressure. There is no evidence that steroids reduce cerebral oedema caused by viral infection and they may exacerbate the infection. Mannitol, though underused, is often very effective.

Treatment of postherpetic neuralgia, once established, is notoriously difficult. There is evidence that amantadine (100 mg twice a day for 28 days) reduces late pain[13]. The drug acts centrally, for it has no effect on DNA viruses. Steroids (for example prednisolone 45 mg daily initially gradually reducing over 28 days) occasionally help[14]. Carbamazepine, even in trigeminal zoster pain, has been disappointing. Unfortunately, in many cases treatment does not work and conventional analgesia must be used. Patients should be reassured that most people will improve with time. In desperate cases we have used thalidomide (100 mg three times a day for 21 days) with occasional success. The action is probably one on the diseased nerve fibres which develop neuropathy and die before normal fibres. The therapeutic margin is narrow and the drug should only be used under hospital supervision.

HERPES SIMPLEX

Invasion of herpes simplex virus (HSV) in the non-immune patient causes 'primary' infection. The virus then lies dormant in the ganglion cells from where it can be intermittently reactivated giving rise to recurrent disease. There are two main types of virus: type I typically invades the skin, the oral mucous membrane and brain, while type II invades the genitalia and newborn. This distinction is not absolute and either type can invade all areas. There is no good cross-protection between the two types although routine serological tests cannot distinguish between them.

Epidemiology

Primary infection is usually a disease of the young but surveys have shown a steady decline in prevalence of antibody to herpes simplex virus. Only about 20–25% of Oxford clinical students have evidence of past infection. This means that in the future, primary herpes simplex virus may become more common in the elderly, when once it was rare.

Herpes simplex virus is spread by close contact with infected people, often venereally or by kissing; medical personnel can become infected by simply handling bodily secretions without wearing protective gloves.

Primary Infection

Primary infection with herpes simplex virus is unusual in the elderly, but when it does occur it is likely to be more severe than in younger patients.

Any part of the integument is at risk from infection. Sites in young adults include the mouth, genitalia, fingers, cheeks and the eye. Presumably non-immune older patients may also develop infection at any of these sites: the risk will depend on their personal habits. After an incubation period of a few days, the infection consists of a local lesion and local adenitis together with constitutional symptoms of fever, malaise, myalgia, arthralgia and some-times generalized lymphadenopathy and splenomegaly. The more general-ized simplex infections are described below.

Acute gingivostomatitis begins with soreness of the mouth and throat. After 1 or 2 days, small rounded vesicles develop on the mucous membrane, tongue, lips, palate and pharynx. The lesions are often very painful and, if untreated, heal after 14–21 days, and virus is excreted for at least 3 weeks. The differential diagnosis includes zoster of the maxillary division of the trigeminal nerve, enteroviruses, beta-haemolytic streptococcus, severe 'aphthous ulcers' and Stevens–Johnson syndrome. Rarely, Epstein–Barr virus, cytomegalovirus and chickenpox can cause confusion. Herpetic whit-lows are reasonably common in the non-immune who nurse ill patients. The finger swells and is very painful, taking several weeks to heal if left untre-ated; the condition is made worse and takes longer to heal if it is incised. It can be confused with bacterial whitlows, normally due to staphylococcus, and orf. Genital herpes in the male appears on the glans penis, coronal sulcus or on the shaft of the penis. Females suffer more with painful labia, vagina and painful micturition. Other venereal diseases should be looked for. Herpes simplex presenting at other sites may be confused with zoster, but zoster, for all practical purposes, never recurs in the same place.

Patients with eczema or Darier's disease have an extensive herpes simplex virus rash (eczema herpeticum) most prominent at the sites of the pre-existing skin lesions. They have a severe systemic illness, and if left untreated have an appreciable mortality. The skin rash has been mistaken for smallpox or eczema vaccinatum. Such patients are at risk from severe recurrent attacks with fever, malaise and local adenitis.

Diagnosis

Primary herpes simplex virus in the elderly is likely to be a difficult diagnosis and vesicular fluid should be collected. Electron microscopy will immedi-ately demonstrate particles typical of the herpes group in general and culture in tissue culture will allow species identification usually within 24 hours. A four-fold rise in titres to herpes simplex virus antibody in paired sera 10 days apart is also diagnostic.

Recurrent Illness

About one in three of patients in their early 20s with antibody to herpes simplex virus gets recurrences regardless of race or country of origin. It is unclear whether recurrences are rarer with increasing age but it seems that older patients complain less. The location of the recurrence follows the primary site of infection. There are often prodromal symptoms; in one survey of healthy patients of all ages[15], 3.4% complained of itching, 27% of tingling and 37% of pain before the vesicles appeared. Trigger features include upper respiratory tract infections (29%), fatigue (17%), emotional stress (15%), physical trauma (12%) and exposure to sunlight (10%) and other forms of ultraviolet light. The common final provoking factor is probably hyperaemia round the ganglion. High fever is a well-known trigger and is not specific to the traditional diseases of pneumococcal pneumonia and malaria. Untreated lesions heal in 6–12 days and the virus can be easily isolated in the first 5 days. In a few patients, each recurrence is followed after about a week by erythema multiforme.

All patients have neutralizing antibody to the virus at the onset of the illness and antibody titres only rarely rise during recurrences. Although it is widely believed that recurrent cold sores always occur in the same place, once infected the nerve is destroyed and so cannot be reinfected. Recurrences may therefore gradually move from place to place.

Eye Infections

Primary infections consist of follicular conjunctivitis with associated adenitis, and the inflammation sometimes spreads forming small corneal opacities. The subsequent recurrences provide a major problem of herpes simplex virus keratitis causing dendritic ulceration and stromal keratitis. Inappropriate treatment with topical steroids will aggravate the lesions and is a not uncommon cause of blindness. Treatment must be supervised by ophthalmologists or others skilled in the use of antiviral chemotherapy.

The differential diagnosis includes infection due to bacteria (in particular *Staph. aureus*) and other viruses (such as adenovirus and rhinovirus) and allergic conjunctivitis. The diagnosis can be confirmed by culture of a conjunctival swab.

Infections of the Central Nervous System

Herpes Simplex Virus Meningitis

Herpes simplex virus meningitis is a benign disease and presents as a lymphocytic meningitis. The virus is only rarely isolated from the CSF and the diagnosis is made retrospectively on a four-fold or greater rise in herpes simplex virus antibody titre in the cerebrospinal fluid.

Herpes Simplex Encephalitis

This is a serious illness with a high mortality and morbidity. It is usually but not invariably a primary infection with an incidence of about 2 per million per year. The illness presents with a short history of high fever (40–41 °C) refractory to antipyretics, severe headache and personality changes. After a few days the patient may fit, develop neck stiffness or focal neurological signs, often including dysphasia, and then lapse into coma. The mortality of untreated patients is about 70%.

The differential diagnosis includes other causes of encephalitis; brain abscesses or intracranial tumours should be excluded by computerized tomography. The diagnosis can be confirmed retrospectively by a four-fold or greater rise in serum herpes simplex virus antibody or more specifically by demonstrating intrathecal herpes simplex virus antibody production. The ratio of antibody in the CSF compared to the serum should be greater than four times the ratio of other proteins. A rapid diagnosis can only be made by detecting antigen directly from a brain biopsy, but the method has a 25% false-negative rate in some hands, probably because the specimen taken was too small.

In a recent study[16] 127 patients were suspected clinically of having herpes simplex virus encephalitis after examination of the cerebrospinal fluid, electroencephalography and computerized tomography. The diagnosis of herpes simplex virus encephalitis was confirmed in 40%, no firm diagnosis was made in 30%, and the final 30% had diagnoses of alcoholic encephalopathy, cerebrovascular disease, other viruses (Epstein–Barr, rubella, cytomegalovirus and influenza) or bacteria (listeria and *Citrobacter freundii*). The study compared the efficacy of 10 days treatment with vidarabine and acyclovir; treatment with acyclovir resulted in the lowest mortality in herpes simplex virus encephalitis (33%). More important, the incidence of severe sequelae was also reduced (see Table 10.1). Management should include intensive care and treatment to lower intracranial pressure.

Table 10.1 Treatment with acyclovir and vidarabine

	Acyclovir	Vidarabine	
All ages (aged 61–76)	27 (12)	26 (9)	
Died	5	12	($p = 0.04$)
Severe sequelae	4	7	
Moderate sequelae	3	2	
Well	15	3	($p = 0.002$)

In view of these results and the lack of side-effects of acyclovir, it seems sensible to treat immediately any patient who may have herpes encephalitis with intravenous acylovir 10 mg/kg 8-hourly given over at least 1 hour until a firm diagnosis is made.

Generalized Herpes Simplex Infections

Severe generalized disease is uncommon in the immunocompetent but there are regular case reports of severe disease in adults. It is sometimes unclear whether the disease is a primary infection or an aggressive reactivation. In severe disease, there is a variable degree of generalized lymphadenopathy together with high fever (38–40 °C), leukopenia, thrombocytopenia and occasionally atypical mononuclear cells with a negative test for heterophil antibodies. Mild hepatitis with raised transaminase is not unusual. Occasionally, adult herpes simplex virus presents as a frank hepatitis which may be fatal. The diagnosis is sometimes suggested by the appearance of typical vesicular lesions, although occasionally oesophagitis is the only extrahepatic manifestation of the disease.

Pneumonitis

Herpes simplex virus pneumonitis was thought to be rare but, since the advent of specific treatment, it is being increasingly recognized[17]. It has been described in burns patients and patients with endotracheal intubations who have squamous metaplasia of the respiratory epithelium. Most cases, however, are described in intensely immunosuppressed patients who develop cold sores; they develop focal or multifocal pneumonitis. A diffuse infiltration is more common following genital herpes. Pneumonitis presents with cough, breathlessness and fever; the patient is hypoxic but only a few pulmonary crackles may be heard on auscultation.

The diagnosis is difficult to establish; lung biopsy with culture, histological examination and examination of tissue for herpes simplex virus antigen by immunofluorescence should be done if a definite diagnosis is needed. Serology is unhelpful and isolation of herpes simplex virus from mucocutaneous sites in the presence of pneumonia is not specific. However, herpes simplex virus pneumonia should be considered in any patient with severe burns, with an endotracheal tube, or who is immunosuppressed with extensive mucocutaneous herpes simplex virus who develops either focal or diffuse lung infiltrates, especially in the presence of tracheitis or oesophagitis.

Management

Herpes labialis is the most common herpes problem in geriatric practice. Patients normally present to geriatricians with other complaints and their cold sore is normally an incidental problem. The easiest management is to use topical idoxuridine (35%) dissolved in dimethylsulphoxide (DMSO) applied five times a day for not more than 3 days (for after that the skin begins to macerate) and to watch the lesion carefully. If there is any sign of progression or if the patient is immunosuppressed then treatment should be switched to oral acyclovir (200 mg five times a day for 7 days)[18]. The drug seems to be well tolerated and there are no absolute contraindications. As yet resistance to acyclovir is not a clinical problem.

Completely well patients who have recurrent cold sores should not be given regular acyclovir, and topical idoxuridine, given early, should be sufficient. In a few cases, recurrences are very severe, or give rise to erythema multiforme, and then acyclovir should be given as early as possible, preferably during the prodromal stage. There is at the moment no clear indication for the use of topical acyclovir, outside the eye; it is not proved to be better than idoxuridine and it is unsound therapeutic policy to apply a drug topically which has an important systemic role.

The best regime for the treatment of uncomplicated primary herpes simplex is still unclear. Intravenous acyclovir is undoubtedly very effective in reducing symptoms and increasing the speed of healing. There is as yet no definite proof that this treatment reduces the incidence of recurrences, although the idea that early intensive viricidal treatment reduces recurrence is attractive. Oral treatment (acyclovir 200 mg five times a day for 7 days) is also effective in reducing symptoms but sometimes the patient finds swallowing difficult.

The management of severe herpes simplex virus infection has been revolutionized by the advent of acyclovir. It seems to be a safe drug free from any severe side-effects, provided it is not given as a bolus (see above under management of zoster, p. 183), and extraordinarily effective against the virus. For most severe infections intravenous acyclovir (5 mg/kg/8-hourly given over 1 hour) for 7 days is sufficient and can be extended if necessary. The dose should be reduced in the presence of impaired renal function. Herpes simplex encephalitis and pneumonitis should be treated early, on clinical suspicion, without waiting for a definite diagnosis.

References

1. Ragozzino, M. W., Melton, L. J., Kurland, L. T., Chu Pin, P. H. and Perry, H. O. (1982a). Risk of cancer after herpes zoster. A population based study. *N. Engl. J. Med.*, **307**, 393–7
2. Ragozzino, M. W., Melton, L. J., Kurland, L. T., Chu, P. H. C. P. and Perry, H. L. O. (1982b). Population-based study of herpes-zoster and its sequelae. *Medicine*, **61**, 310–16

3. Weller, T. H. (1983). Varicella and herpes zoster. Changing concepts of the natural history, control and importance of a not-so-benign virus. *N. Engl. J. Med.*, **309,** 1362–8; 1434–40

4. Womack, L. W. and Liesegang, T. J. (1983). Complications of herpes zoster ophthalmicus. *Arch. Ophthalmol.*, **101,** 42–5

5. Jemsek, J., Greenberg, S. B., Taber, L., Harvey, D., Gershon, A. and Couch, R. B. (1983). Herpes zoster-associated encephalitis: clinicopathologic report of 12 cases and review of the literature. *Medicine,* **62,** 81–97

6. Dolin, R. (1978). Herpes zoster-varicella infections in the immunosuppressed patients *Ann. Intern. Med.*, **89,** 375–88

7. Mazur, M. H. and Dolin, R. (1978). Herpes zoster at the NIH: A 20-year experience. *Am. J. Med.*, **65,** 738–44

8. Juel-Jensen, B. E. and MacCallum, F. O. (1972). *Herpes Simplex Varicella and Zoster: Clinical Manifestations and Treatment.* (London: William Heinemann Medical Books Ltd.)

9. Balfour, H. H., Bean, B., Laskin, O. L., Ambinder, R. F., Meyers, J. D., Wade, J. C., Zaia, J. A., Aeppli, D., Kirk, L. E., Segreti, A. C., Keeney, R. E. and the Burroughs Wellcome Collaborative acyclovir study group (1983). Acyclovir halts progression of herpes zoster in immunocompromised patients. *N. Engl. J. Med.*, **308,** 1448–53

10. Bean, B., Braun, C. and Balfour, H. H. (1982). Acyclovir therapy for acute herpes zoster. *Lancet,* **2,** 118–21

11. Juel-Jensen, B. E., Khan, J. A. and Pasvol, G. (1983). High-dose intravenous acyclovir in the treatment of zoster: a double-blind placebo-controlled trial. *J. Inf.,* **6,** Suppl. 1, 31–6

12. Shigeta, S., Yokota, T., Iwabuchi, T., Baber, M., Konno, K., Oqata, M. and De Clercq, E. (1983). Comparative efficacy of anit-herpes drugs against various strains of varicella-zoster virus. *J. Infect. Dis.,* **147,** 576–84

13. Galbraith, A. W. (1983). Prevention of post-herpetic neuralgia by amantadine hydrochloride (Symmetrel). *Br. J. Clin. Pract.,* **37,** 304–6

14. Keckes, K. and Basher, A. M. (1980). Do corticosteroids prevent post-herpetic neuralgia? *Br. J. Dermatol.,* **102,** 551–5

15. Bader, C., Crumpacker, C. S., Schnipper, L. E., Ransil, B., Clark, J. E., Arndt, E. and Freedberg, M. (1978). The natural history of recurrent facial-oral infection with herpes simplex virus. *J. Infect. Dis.,* **138,** 897–905

16. Skoldenberg, B., Forsgren, F., Alestig, K., Bergstrom, T., Burman, L., Dahlqvist, Anders, F., Fryden, A., Lovgren, K., Norlin, K., Norrby, R., Olding-Stengvist, E., Stiernstedt, G., Uhnoo, I. and De Vahl, K. (1984). Acyclovir versus vidarabine in herpes simplex encephalitis. *Lancet,* **2,** 707–11

17. Ramsey, P. G., Fife, K. H., Hackman, C., Meyers, J. D. and Corey, L. (1982). Herpes simplex virus pneumonia. Clinical, virologic, and pathologic features in 20 patients. *Ann. Intern. Med.,* **97,** 813–20

18. Nilsen, A. E., Aasen, T., Halsos, A. M., Kingw, B. R., Tiotta, E. A. L., Wikstrom, K. and Fiddian, A. P. (1982). Efficacy of oral acyclovir in the treatment of initial and recurrent genital herpes. *Lancet,* **2,** 571–7

11

Opportunistic Infections

B. MOORE-SMITH

DEFINITIONS

In 1956 *Blakiston's Gould Medical Dictionary*, 3rd Edition defined opportunistic thus: 'In bacteriology: an organism incapable of inducing disease in a healthy host, but able to produce infections in a less resistant or injured host . . .'. By 1981 *Dorland's Illustrated Medical Dictionary*, 26th Edition had softened the rigid 'incapable' to 'does not ordinarily cause': 'denoting a micro-organism which does not ordinarily cause disease but which under certain circumstances (e.g. impaired immune responses), becomes pathogenic'.

Common to both definitions is the concept of micro-organisms whose infectivity is low but which grasp their chance when the potential host is for some reason less resistant or injured. The advances in immunology over the 25-year period colour the later definition, but in the elderly this may serve only to distract attention from much more common breaches of host defences by invasive therapy through the use of intravenous lines, catheters or intratracheal airways.

The *Merck Manual* 1977, 13th Edition, perhaps has the most balanced view: 'Infections ranging from minor to fatal, caused by normally non-pathogenic organisms in patients whose host defence mechanisms have been compromised'. The range of outcomes 'from minor to fatal' is worth emphasizing in the elderly whose opportunistic infections are less commonly associated with the major blood dyscrasias or massive therapeutic immunosuppressive manoeuvres so frequently the cause of such infections in younger age groups and in them so often fatal.

191

PREDISPOSING FACTORS

Introduction

In elderly people, compromise of host defence mechanisms holds the key to the majority of opportunistic infections. However, factors predisposing to these infections may include, as well as defects in surface defences, instances as diverse as: alterations in immune function with age, malnutrition, pre-existing primary infections, antibiotic treatment, major surgery, renal failure, diabetes, leukaemias and lymphomas, immunocompromise and immunosuppression, the AIDS syndrome, and institutionalization. Those aspects of particular relevance to the elderly will be discussed.

Surface Defences

The elderly human being, as in earlier years, wages a permanent defensive battle against the micro-organisms which assail him. The front line of the battle lies on the skin which, like the battlements of old, is pierced by openings for entry and exit. However well defended, such breaches inevitably offer the opportunity for attack from without, and relatively weak attackers may force an entry if the defences are weakened. It is ironic that some modern therapeutic manoeuvres may assist the attack of micro-organisms by bypassing the defences.

The Skin and its Orifices

Normal skin offers highly effective protection even in old age although its continuity then may be more easily broken by minor trauma. Other breaches can be caused by burns and by ulceration such as leg ulcers or bedsores.

Normal orifices of the skin include the eyes, ears, nose, mouth, anus, urethra and vagina. Decreased secretion of tears (Sjögren's syndrome), or inability to fully close the eyelids (facial palsy) predispose to infection; however, otitis externa is surprisingly uncommon despite often major accumulations of wax in the external meatus. With an intact tympanic membrane, middle ear disease arising *de novo* in old age is rare.

The nose and mouth are obvious portals through which infections, both common and opportunistic, may gain entry. The upper gastrointestinal tract is relatively inhospitable to most micro-organisms but in the lower respiratory passages the susceptibility of the normal protecting and cleansing mechanism (the upward-moving, cilia-carried, mucus secretion) to inhibition by influenza viruses, or damage by bronchitis, is well known. Secondary infection by common, or less common agents, such as pulmonary aspergillosis, often follows.

The lower gastrointestinal tract is usually well protected by its resident bacterial flora from attack but this very flora, especially bacteroides and *Clostridium septicum,* may gain entry through neoplastic ulceration and lead to left perinephric abscess as a mark of unsuspected malignancy of the large bowel[1]. The long male urethra flushed by urine is an effective defence but the short female urethra and the vagina, by now devoid of its low pH defence induced by lactobacilli, are much more prone to invasion.

While the mechanical defences of the skin are for the most part very effective, modern invasive therapeutic manoeuvres may compromise them unwittingly even though the intervention itself may be lifesaving. Thus intravenous cannulation, central venous pressure monitoring lines and temporary transcutaneous cardiac pacemakers all breach the integrity of the skin through which they pass and offer a route of access for micro-organisms which may indeed have their passage to the central parts of the circulation greatly eased. That such opportunities are only infrequently the source of major infection is a tribute to the host's other defence mechanisms as well as to a good aseptic technique on insertion and to subsequent care. Careful assessment of the need for such intervention is always necessary.

A body orifice is an open invitation to the insertion of some form of channel. Thus the nose and the oesophagus carrying the ubiquitous nasogastric tube, the trachea (whether affording entry to an oral endotracheal tube, or to a tracheostomy and its associated external airways), and notably the urethra are all intubated or catheterized, if not with abandon, sometimes without full realization of the potential consequences. The outer defences having been bypassed, the host is forced back on to its second and remarkably sophisticated lines of resistance, those of the humoral and cellular defences which form the immune system.

ALTERATIONS IN IMMUNE FUNCTION WITH AGE

Non-specific Cellular and Humoral Defences

A detailed description of immune defence mechanisms has been given in Chapter 2. In outline it will be recalled that from antiquity the mechanical barriers referred to above have been supplemented by the non-specific phagocytic cell system: in man represented by the tissue histiocytes, the fixed macrophages of liver, spleen and lymph nodes and by the circulating monocytes and polymorphonuclear leukocytes. In addition to their phagocytic function macrophages play an important role in the specific immune response to infection.

There is a further natural (non-specific), as opposed to adaptive (specific) humoral defence mechanism: that of the complement system. Present in serum this system's proteolytic enzyme sequential cascade may be triggered either by direct contact with some bacteria, the 'alternative' (and probably more primitive) pathway, or by contact with immobilized antibody, the 'classical' pathway. In either case the result is the formation of a 'membrane attack complex' which attaches to cell or bacterial membranes and causes lysis of the cell or organism.

Evidence for, and the effects of, deficiencies in the elderly in the phagocytic and complement systems and the humoral and cell-mediated immune systems will be considered.

The Phagocytic Cell Systems in the Elderly

There are two cell populations exhibiting phagocytosis: the related tissue macrophages and peripheral blood monocytes, and the polymorphonuclear leukocytes.

Macrophages and Monocytes

There is no evidence that macrophage numbers alter with advancing age but there is no information about monocytes[2]. There is some evidence that macrophages are already activated in old age and are more efficient at phagocytosis[3], but this is accompanied by a decrease in antigen-processing efficiency[4]. Overall there is no evidence that changes in macrophage function are implicated in altered defences to infection[2]. This is especially relevant as macrophages are particularly important in defence against some facultative intracellular parasites, many of which may behave opportunistically.

Polymorphonuclear leukocytes

Neutrophil adherence, an important component of the inflammatory response, is reported to be elevated in the elderly over the age of 80, especially in women[5]. The same authors found 13% of healthy over-80s to have impaired polymorph chemotaxis. On the other hand yeast phagocytosis was not impaired[5] although others have found decreased phagocytosis[6]. The results of tests of neutrophil antimicrobial activity are variable, but any deficiences observed may be related to impaired neutrophil metabolic function noted in persons over the age of 70[7].

Certain infections, such as staphylococcal, are more prevalent and severe in the elderly[8] and may be related to neutrophil dysfunction. Interestingly neutrophils secrete endogenous pyrogen, and if this is deficient it might explain the often muted pyrexial response to infection in the elderly.

All in all there is some evidence of impaired neutrophil function in the elderly which may in part explain the increased incidence of infection in the elderly especially in institutional settings[9].

The Complement System

In a system as complex as this, deficiencies of its individual parts are to be expected and indeed C2, C3, C5, C6, C7 and C9 deficiency states have all been described[10]. They are rare, some are associated with increased susceptibility to bacterial infection, notably deficiencies of C3, which is a key part of both major complement pathways. Patients with C5, C6, C7 and C8 deficiencies are particularly susceptible to meningococcal or gonococcal infection[11] but there is no evidence currently available to suggest that failure of part or parts of the complement system plays any major role in opportunistic infection in the elderly. Indeed Phair *et al.*[8] noted, but could not explain, elevation of C3 and properdin levels in their aged subjects (mean age 76).

Specific Humoral and Cellular Defences

The second line of defence, modern in evolutionary terms – the specific immune response in man – has two parts: (1) humoral (antibody production) which depends on B lymphocytes with help from macrophages and T lymphocytes; and (2) cell-mediated responses dependent on T lymphocytes.

The humoral (antibody) response is very effective against extracellular micro-organisms, while micro-organisms which are intracellular during the infective process (such as viruses, mycobacteria, brucella, listeria), are protected from antibody, and cell-mediated responses are more important in defence against them. These latter responses are mediated by T lymphocytes of which there are (at least) four types: cytotoxic T cells – key cells in virus immunity; helper T cells – essential for most antibody responses; suppressor T cells – they inhibit both B and T cell responses; delayed hypersensitivity T cells – they attract and activate a variety of cells. Other T cell functions include: cytotoxicity, production of lymphokines which control macrophage activity and viral reproduction, and also the production of transfer factor and the lysis of viral infected cells.

The Adaptive Humoral System

This is characterized by the production of specific antibodies, the immunoglobulins. There are four main classes: IgA, IgG, IgM and IgE. Antibody deficiency syndromes are uncommon and are related to abnormalities of various lymphocytes which produce the immunoglobulins. The better known syndromes include X-linked hypogammaglobulinaemia, seen in children between 6 months and 2 years of age; late-onset hypogamma-globulinaemia which may occur from 1 to 70 years of age but is commonest in the third decade, and thymoma with hypogammaglobulinaemia occurring between 40 and 70 years.

In the first there are no circulating mature B cells, and T cells contain enzyme abnormalities compatible with immaturity, while all the serum immunoglobulin classes are almost unrecordable. In the late onset variety, 30% are lymphocytopenic, B cells are few in 25% and absent in another 25%, and only IgM can be found in any quantity on *in vitro* testing. In the thymoma-related variety the hypogammaglobulinaemia is moderate and salivary IgA usually maintained.

None of these syndromes is common; the first two usually present early in life and the third in middle age, despite the considerable evidence of mounting abnormalities of the immune systems as age advances.

Paralleling thymic involution, circulating levels of natural antibody decline with age as does the antigen-induced primary antibody response in experimental animals[12]. However, the secondary response appears unimpaired in old age. It is the T cell-dependent responses that decline with age, T cell-independent responses being unaffected[13]. There is evidence that at least in animals, some antibody produced may have lessened avidity[12]. In man the evidence is conflicting, some studies showing normal response to vaccination in old age, others the reverse, but some of the populations studied were of already dependent and disabled individuals. Overall, in man there is little evidence of clinically important abnormalities of antibody production with age which might contribute to opportunistic infection.

Cell-Mediated Immunity

There are two aspects of this part of the immune system: the cells themselves and their function. Much of the evidence is summarized by Fox[14].

Stem Cells

Bone marrow stem cells remain haemopoietically normal in development and function throughout life and their numbers increase with age. However, their immune functions deteriorate: they are less able to home to the thymus, essential for their maturation; the rate of formation of B cells falls; their ability to repair X-ray induced damage decreases and their potential for transplantation diminishes.

Lymphocytes and their Subsets

As a total class their actual numbers are probably little changed with age though opinions vary. More important are the relative proportions of various subsets and their functions.

T Lymphocytes – The evidence concerning overall T cell numbers is conflicting but old T lymphocytes show membrane, cytoplasm and organelle abnormalities.

Suppressor T Cells – Techniques involving the use of monoclonal antibodies show a decrease in the percentage and number of suppressor T cells or at least of some suppressor sub-varieties. The other T cell subsets are unaffected by age and the T cell helper-cell percentage and numbers in particular do not change, nor does their function as far as is known. Suppressor T cell function declines with age exponentially and enhances the production of autoantibodies but not of antibodies to foreign antigens. The increase of antibodies appears to be a marker of declining T cell function more than of disease.

B Lymphocytes – Their numbers increase with age, but the rise in monoclonal gammopathies with age suggests B cell qualitative changes which have been confirmed in both humans and mice.

Bacterial endotoxins, acting as polyclonal activators of B cells, favour the development of B cells devoted to the production of autoantibodies to the detriment of antibody production to foreign antigens. In this connection the rate of Gram-negative bacterial oropharyngeal colonization increases in the frail elderly and might well be a potent source of polyclonal activation responsible for a decline in immune response to foreign antigens from other infections. It is also known that bacterial endotoxin has an anti-inflammatory effect[15]. These are matters clearly of much interest.

Age Effects on Cell-Mediated Immunity

In vitro studies have shown decreased responsiveness of T cells to stimulation, and a decreased reproductive ability, for example, 92% of lymphocytes from young subjects had divided at least once after 72 hours in culture, in contrast to only 70% of lymphocytes from older subjects.

B cell responses to anti-Ig antibody increase with age in relation to a loss of inhibitory cells; so also do their T cell-dependent responses, probably related to suppressor T cell loss with age. Perhaps not surprisingly in so complex a field, *in vivo* tests have produced conflicting evidence. These changes are linked with a correlation between anergy and increased mortality, though which of the anergy or the increased mortality is cause and which effect is uncertain. However, tuberculin-negative elderly individuals are very susceptible to tuberculosis and waning immunity seems to be a factor as it does also in the increased risk of shingles in the elderly[16].

In summary, the waning influence of the thymus with age affects the function of the subsets of T cells. Both helper T cell function which controls some antibody production by B cells, and suppressor T cell function which can inhibit T and B cell responses, are depressed in old age. The clinical results are a deterioration of the primary antibody response, an increased production of autoantibodies and some waning of cell-mediated immunity. The increased morbidity and mortality from infection in senescence are probably directly linked to these changes, which in turn may be experienced in a variety of clinical situations.

MALNUTRITION AND INFECTIONS

Previously it has been assumed that in developed countries malnutrition in the elderly, in the sense of undernutrition, was chiefly due to environmental and social factors and that these led to ill-health. Over the last 20 years or so it has become apparent that this is rarely the case[17]. Rather is the reverse true: when malnutrition is diagnosed underlying disease is usually found to account for it, and the marked decline in nutrient intake with age is due in the main to the rising incidence of physical and mental disability, and rarely to social or environmental factors alone.

The most consistent clinical effect of malnutrition, whether acquired primarily or secondarily, is impairment of immune responses and an increase in the susceptibility to, and severity of, most infections[18]. There is reason to think that T cells fail to mature as a result of deficiency of the zinc-rich thymic hormone. In turn T cells fail to produce lymphokines which activate mononuclear phagocytes to destroy intracellular pathogens such as *Mycobacterium tuberculosis, Salmonella typhi* or *Toxoplasma gondii*. Humoral defences also, for example, complement fractions, except C4, and specific immunoglobulins, may be affected by protein deficiency. Both complement pathways may be severely depressed in states of malnutrition and their constituents then exhibit a drop in the face of infection instead of the usual rise. Chemotaxis, opsonization and microbicidal activities may all be affected by protein deficiency.

Functional immune system defects are well defined in malnutrition for T lymphocytes and the complement cascade with a consequent increased susceptibility to intracellular pathogens and Gram-negative sepsis. Trace element deficiencies of iron, zinc, copper and selenium may well be important also in depressing cell-mediated immunities.

In short, while malnutrition is frequently the result of underlying disease, rather than of social or environmental factors, it may have important effects on the host's ability to resist infection and hence open the way to opportunistic pathogens as well as the more commonly experienced organisms.

PRE-EXISTING INFECTION

A pre-existing infection can result in abnormal and damaging responses especially in viral and intracellular bacterial infections. Among such responses are autoimmune reactions and immune complex deposition: the latter may well be a more common cause of 'second bout fever' and skin rashes than the commonly blamed allergy to antibiotics.

While infections such as measles or infectious mononucleosis are extremely rare in the elderly in westernized societies, the relatively recent recognition of the acquired immunodeficiency syndrome (AIDS), probably due to the retrovirus, human T lymphocyte virus, type III[19] is of considerable interest. One feature of AIDS is Kaposi's sarcoma whose incidence formerly was best known in Italians and in Jews of Central European origin in their sixth and seventh decades. Another important feature is the incidence of opportunistic infection due to T helper cell lymphopenia and an inverted helper: suppressor T cell ratio. *Pneumocystis carinii*, toxoplasmosis, cytomegalovirus and cryptosporidiosis are the commonest opportunistic organisms in this setting. The relationship of these two major features of this syndrome to depleted immune reactions is striking, and what might be regarded as the apparent ageing effect of a virus infection is of great interest.

ANTIBIOTIC TREATMENT

Treatment with broad-spectrum antibiotics, especially in combination, or even narrow-spectrum antibiotics in massive or prolonged dosage, is well known to cause difficulties in relation to alteration of the normal body flora of micro-organisms. The problem was clearly enunciated as long ago as 1959 by Finland *et al.*[20], who remarked that broad-spectrum antibiotic usage seemed to enhance the number, pathogenicity and invasiveness of various micro-organisms which under ordinary circumstances appeared rather benign – as nice a definition of opportunism as one could wish for.

The elderly, for reasons already alluded to, are prone to infection and, therefore, liable to be treated with antibiotics. The unwanted effects include colonization of the respiratory tract by enterobacilli which may be only transient, but in the gastrointestinal tract the alteration of flora to that of antibiotic-resistant organisms may persist for months or even years. In addition, Gram-negative bacteria have the ability to transmit plasmids, carrying R factors for antibiotic resistance, to previously non-resistant organisms.

One result of such altered flora is superinfection (invasion by organisms resistant to the antibiotic being given). Such superinfections occur, often on the fourth or fifth day of treatment, especially at the extremes of life, in those with chronic infections or other debilitating diseases, during courses in excessive dosage of single antimicrobials, or of combinations of broad-spectrum antibiotics. They may convert a benign, self-limiting disease to a serious, prolonged or fatal outcome. The organisms most involved include Gram-negative enterobacilli, fungi and resistant staphylococci.

THE PATIENT WITH ACQUIRED IMMUNODEFICIENCY

Individuals with primary immunodeficiencies, such as agammaglobulinaemia, or DiGeorge's syndrome, are unlikely to survive into old age but there is a wide range of conditions which predisposes to some degree of secondary immune incompetence. The current outbreak of the acquired immunodeficiency syndrome although of great theoretical and, indeed, practical, interest is as yet not a clinical problem in the elderly. However, a substantial proportion of elderly hospital in-patients exhibit a combination of risk factors which may lead to immune deficiencies. The attacks on surface defences, the alterations in immune processes with age, the place of malnutrition, the role of pre-existing infection, and the problems engendered by antibiotic treatment have already been referred to.

The multifactorially ill elderly patient may frequently suffer from diabetes. While contrary to general belief, diabetics are no more susceptible to staphylococcal infection, postoperative wound infection, or nosocomial infection than other patients, they are much more prone to candida vulvovaginitis, gingivitis, urinary tract infections (particularly in elderly women) and foot ulcers. They also are more prone to septic shock syndromes and gas-forming infections[21]. The reasons, at least in part, lie in the alterations in cell-mediated immunity and disturbed polymorph activity seen mostly in insulin-dependent diabetics. There is, however, little information in relation to elderly diabetics who are usually not insulin-dependent.

Many elderly patients have a reduced renal reserve and are chronically uraemic. Suppression of immune responsiveness and depressed numbers of circulating lymphocytes were noted 20 years ago in uraemia[22].

Surgical operations, even in healthy individuals[23], induce depletion of all types of circulating lymphocytes and a state of immunosuppression quite apart from the inevitable breaching of tissue planes. Splenectomy, which may have been carried out years before, leaves the patient with defective immunoglobulin production, delayed macrophage mobilization and some antibody deficiencies[24]. They are more prone to infection, especially pneumococcal.

Another important group of elderly patients with major defects in their defences against infection include those with malignant diseases, especially acute non-lymphocytic leukaemias in which anatomical barriers may be broken. Antibiotics may alter the normal flora, nutrition is often poor, both cell-mediated and humoral immunity may be altered, and neutropenia, due to either disease or its therapy, is so frequently the primary risk factor.

Lymphomas lead to altered cell-mediated immunity with abnormal delayed hypersensitivity and T cell responses. Again neutropenia may be the result of therapy. Multiple myeloma is not infrequently seen in the elderly and produces B cell defects with decreased immunoglobulin production.

Solid tumours are, of course, very common in elderly patients, but although the cell-mediated immune response is often altered it does not seem to form a significant risk factor for infection.

There is also the group of patients whose immune responses have been compromised by therapy. While systemic lupus erythematosus (SLE) and polyarteritis are relatively uncommon in the elderly, rheumatoid arthritis is frequent and giant cell arteritis often seen. Although drugs such as cyclophosphamide and azathioprine are not widely used in their treatment in the elderly, corticosteroids are and have multiple effects on neutrophil, lymphocyte and macrophage functions which manifest as suppression of the inflammatory responses and an increased susceptibility to infection[25,26].

The results of altering defences against infection in the elderly are exemplified in the very differing rates of nosocomial (institutionally acquired) infections in patients aged 65 and over compared with younger age groups. Bram and Torok[9] reported a 10% nosocomial infection rate in those aged over 65 compared with 2.1% under that age. They also reported a change in the organisms chiefly involved, from staphylococci in the 1950s altering from the 1960s onwards to Gram-negative bacilli and fungi. They drew attention to many of the factors referred to above in causing the five-fold increase in the nosocomial infection rate.

OPPORTUNISTIC MICRO-ORGANISMS

Whether an ordinarily pathogenic organism causes an infection depends on the balance between the scale of the invasion and the state of the defences; ordinarily non-pathogenic organisms, however, need a greater breach in the defences to become pathogenic. There is, therefore, no rigid dividing line between the two types but opportunism is suggested by the identity of the organism found in particular circumstances; that is, the identity of the organisms suggests the presence of the defensive breach even though the organism is a common one.

Examples abound in everyday practice; for example *E. coli* found in every colon is the commonest cause of urinary tract infection and not infrequently found in the respiratory tract. *Streptococcus viridans,* a universal commensal in the mouth, is well known as the leading organism to cause infective endocarditis; interestingly in the elderly a wider range of organisms, including Gram-negative species, is implicated due to a combination of a suitable focus, altered immunity and the presence of Gram-negative bacteria already invading other systems.

They are, however, patterns of opportunistic infection which suggest particular defensive deficiences (Table 11.1).

Table 11.1 Defensive deficiencies and patterns of opportunistic infection

Surface deficiencies	Phagocytic deficiencies	Humoral deficiencies	Cellular deficiencies
Staph. aureus	Staph. aureus	Pneumococcus	Viruses: especially herpes viruses, such as cytomegalovirus, herpes simplex, varicella zoster
Pseudomonas	Pseudomonas	Beta-haemolytic streptococcus	
E. coli	E. coli		
Proteus	Klebsiella	H. influenzae	Fungi:
H. influenzae	Candida	Neisseria	Aspergillus
		(Pseudomonas)	Mucor
Klebsiella	+		Cryptococcus
	Mycobacteria		Candida
Candida			Protozoa:
	Nocardia		Pneumocystis carinii
	Legionella		Toxoplasma gondii
			Gram-negative rods
	Listeria		atypical mycobacteria

This table is illustrative rather than comprehensive and while there are clear differences between some groups there is also much overlap. In clinical practice in the elderly it is organisms in the first three groups that are encountered most commonly. Major deficiencies in cell-mediated immunity are usually secondary to the use of immunosuppressive drugs either for the control of conditions such as systemic lupus erythematosus, polyarteritis, hepatitis, nephritis or rheumatoid arthritis, or after organ or bone marrow transplant. Aggressive treatment of these conditions is infrequently practised in the elderly and transplantation is virtually never performed.

In the elderly, as indicated earlier, the isolation of an organism indicating some degree of opportunism is most likely to be due to interference, often therapeutically, with surface defences by, for example, catheters, intravenous lines or transcutaneous cardiac pacemakers, or by burns, bedsores or ulceration. Alterations in immunity, of course, also play a part.

DIAGNOSIS

The similarity between the frail elderly as a group and younger, usually iatrogenically, immunosuppressed patients is nowhere more obvious than in the diagnosis of infection. The problems of diagnosis experienced in such younger patients are of everyday occurrence in the elderly.

Clinically the classical sign of infection, the inflammatory response, is often substantially modified. Pain, especially in the abdomen, may be minimal and guarding and rigidity absent; frank pus may be replaced by a serous exudate, and low-grade fever may be the only overt sign of infection in Gram-negative septicaemia in a hypotensive patient. The presence of a breach of surface defences, such as a urinary catheter or intravenous line, skin ulceration or bedsores, must be noted and general clinical examination must be meticulous. The chest is notoriously difficult to examine in elderly patients and physical signs may be few in the face of major infection and quite obvious X-ray changes. The abdomen is equally subject to covert pathology including sepsis with few abdominal signs[27], free gas under the diaphragm may be seen on an erect abdominal film in a patient with a soft abdomen.

Investigation of suspected infection requires repeated clinical examination, chest and abdominal X-ray films, repeated blood cultures (for such entities as *Streptococcus bovis* endocarditis which may accompany colonic neoplasms, as well as for septicaemia from any source), total and differential white cell count, routine biochemistry (for acute or chronic uraemia, acidotic or alkalotic states or glycosuria), and blood gases as indicated. A simple Gram stain of pus or exudate obtained by appropriate swabbing, or of sputum, may be helpful. If fungal infection is suspected an immediate diagnosis may be obtained from wet mount lactophenol cotton blue or a 10% potassium hydroxide preparation. Meningitis is uncommon in the elderly, clinically or as an unexpected post-mortem finding, but if at all suspected direct CSF microscopy should be performed and include an Indian ink stain and latex slide test agglutination for *Cryptococcus neoformans*.

As always in the elderly a high index of suspicion allied to a low threshold for appropriate investigation is required to avoid unnecessary morbidity and mortality from opportunistic infection.

PROPHYLAXIS

Opportunistic organisms like their more pathogenic relatives are ever-present in the milieu in which elderly patients move. However, they require more of a helping hand to gain access to a host. Part of the help they obtain is by virtue of alterations in the immune systems of elderly patients. There is little in the present state of knowledge that can be done to influence these changes. T-cell stimulating agents such as thymosin (thymic hormone), transfer factor, a lymphokine which enhances cell-mediated immunity, and levamisole, became temporarily popular but offer little practical advantage in the absence of simultaneous antimicrobial therapy. An exception is the use of thymosin in generalized immunodeficiency but this is not a condition seen much in the elderly.

The more fruitful approach to prophylaxis lies in the avoidance of damage to surface defences by good nursing practice to prevent skin trauma, including bedsores, burns and ulceration and especially to ensure adequate hydration. Dehydration may contribute to reduced secretions of many types and consequent infection often by opportunist organisms. Diminished respiratory mucus opens the way to respiratory infection, scanty saliva to parotitis, reduced urinary flow to urinary infection, lessened skin and tissue turgor to cellulitis. Dehydration is a potent cause of confusion which in turn predisposes to many of the above.

Another major cause of damage to surface defences is the widespread use of intravenous or other cannulae for a variety of invasive treatments. Careful appraisal of the indications for such manoeuvres is mandatory, and if the indications are compelling continuing close supervision of the apparatus whether intravenous, nasogastric, intratracheal or transurethral is essential. The difficulties are exemplified by the frequency of urinary infections after catheterization. Thrombophlebitis associated with intravenous lines is commonplace, but fortunately with good care central infection of the cardiovascular system can be largely prevented. In all these instances a balance must be struck between the benefit to the patient of the mode of treatment and the possible hazards.

Antibiotics in Prophylaxis

Mention must also be made of the place of antibiotics in prophylaxis. A normal bacterial flora acts as an effective barrier to invasion; witness the rapid occurrence of mucosal candidiasis during treatment with broad-spectrum antibiotics or the supervention of *Clostridium difficile* in antibiotic-associated pseudomembranous colitis. At one time there was a vogue for total-bowel decontamination in neutropenic patients because of the frequency with which they acquired Gram-negative septicaemia. More latterly it has been preferable to selectively remove the aerobic flora with co-trimoxazole and to leave the anaerobes as protective 'wallpaper' against opportunistic pathogens. The place of antibiotics in prophylaxis is limited except in the context of the prevention of infective endocarditis and septicaemias in relation to dental extractions in the presence of cardiac abnormalities or prostheses, and in the prevention of Gram-negative septicaemia in repeated or difficult male catheterization.

TREATMENT

The principles of treatment of opportunistic infections are straightforward. Treatment should always be with the most specific and least toxic agent available. An attempt should always be made to identify the organism and to determine its sensitivity. Inevitably, in for instance an acute Gram-negative septicaemia following urinary catherization, the urgency may preclude awaiting culture and sensitivity reports and treatment must commence on a 'best guess' basis. Treatment can be modified in the light of later laboratory evidence if the patient fails to respond satisfactorily to the initial choice of therapy.

Drugs of Choice

The most dangerous opportunisitic pathogens are enteric Gram-negative rods and *Pseudomonas aeruginosa*. The most effective drugs are cephalosporins, aminoglycosides and the antipseudomonal penicillins. Current advice[28] favours the combination of an aminoglycoside and a beta-lactamase antibiotic (either a penicillin or a cephalosporin) although there are encouraging reports of single-drug therapy with 'third generation' cephalosporins. The precise choice depends, among other factors, on any previous culture results, the 'local' bacterial resistance pattern and any history of patient allergies.

The drugs currently involved are the penicillins azlocillin and piperacillin, and the cephalosporins cefotaxime and latamoxef. Gentamicin and netilmicin are the aminoglycosides of choice, but great care is necessary in dosage in the face of any degree of renal failure.

Less commonly, elderly patients develop opportunistic mycoses, candidosis, aspergillosis and mucomycosis being the commonest. Amphotericin B, which has numerous side-efects, is the drug of choice in systemic mycoses. It can be combined with flucytosine which should not be used alone because of the development of drug resistance[29].

Disseminated opportunistic viral infections are rare in elderly patients but if they occur herpes simplex and varicella zoster respond well to acyclovir. It is not effective against cytomegalovirus.

CONCLUSION

Opportunistic infection in the elderly is common and is usually dependent on a breach of surface defences. The altering immune status with age is of great theoretical interest, but is of lesser importance in the causation of such infections.

References

1. Keusch, G. T. (1974). Opportunistic infections in colon carcinoma. *Am. J. Clin. Nutr.*, **27**, 1481–1485

2. Puxty, J. A. H. and Fox, R. A. (1984). The phagocytic system. In: Fox R. A. (ed.) *Immunology and Infection in the Elderly*. pp. 322–3. (Edinburgh: Churchill Livingstone)

3. Perkins, E. H. (1971). Phagocytic activity of aged mice. *J. Reticuloendothel. Soc.* **9**, 642–3

4. Legge, J. S. and Austin, C. M. (1968). Antigen localisation and the immune response as a function of age. *Aust. J. Exp. Biol. Med. Sci.*, **46**, 361–5

5. Corberand, J., Noyen, F. and Laharrague, P. (1981). Polymorphonuclear functions and ageing in humans. *J. Am. Geriatr. Soc.*, **29**, 391–7

6. Ivanova, N. I. (1978). Age characteristics of the phagocytic reaction of neutrophils. *Vrachebnoe Delo.*, **5**, 49

7. van Epps, D. E., Goodwin, J. S. and Murphy, S. (1978). Age-dependent variations in polymorphonuclear leucocyte chemiluminescence. *Infect. Immun.*, **22**, 57–61

8. Phair, J. P., Kauffman, E. A., Bjornson, A., Gallagher, J., Adams, L. and Hess, E. V. (1978). Host defences in the aged. Evaluation of components of the inflammatory and immune responses. *J. Inf. Dis.*, **138**, 67–73

9. Brem, A. M. and Torok, E. M. (1979). Nosocomial infections in the elderly. *Hosp. Top. Chicago*, **57(6)**, 10, 40–3

10. Goldstein, I. M. and Marder, S. R. (1983). Infection and hypocomplementaemia. *Ann. Rev. Med.*, **34**, 47–53

11. Frank, M. M. (1979). The complement system in host defence and inflammation. *Rev. Inf. Dis.*, **1(3)**, 483–501

12. Fox, R. A. (1984). The effect of ageing on the immune response. In: Fox R. A. (ed) *Immunology and Infection in the Elderly*. pp. 297–8. (Edinburgh: Churchill Livingstone)

13. Smith, A. M. (1976). The effects of age on the immune response to type III pneumococcal polysaccharide and bacterial lipopolysaccharide in BALB/C, SJL/J and C3H mice. *J. Immunol.*, **116**, 469–74

14. Fox, R. A. (1984). The effect of ageing on the immune response. In: Fox R. A. (ed) *Immunology and Infection in the Elderly*. pp. 294–7. (Edinburgh: Churchill Livingstone)

15. Verghese, M. W. and Snyderman, R. (1981). Differential anti-inflammatory effects of L.P.S. in susceptible and resistant mouse strains. *J. Immunol.*, **127**, 288–93

16. Miller, A. E. (1980). Selective decline in cellular immune response to varicella-zoster in the elderly. *Neurology*, **30**, 582–7

17. Exton-Smith, A. N. (1973). Changing views on nutrition of the elderly. *The Glaxo Volume*, **38**, 15–26

18. Keûsch, G. T. (1982). Nutrition and infections. *Comprehensive Ther.*, **12(1)**, 10–14

19. Chiengsong-Popov, R., Weiss, R. A., Dalgleish, A., Tedder, R. A., Jeffries, D. J., Shanson, D. C., Ferns, R. B., Briggs, E. M., Weller, I. V. D., Mitton, S., Adler, M. W., Farthing, C., Lawrence, A. G., Gazzard, B. G., Weber, J., Harris, J. R. W., Pinching, A. J., Craske, J. and Barbara, J. A. J. (1984). Prevalence of antibody to human T-lymphotropic virus type III in AIDS and AIDS-risk patients in Britain. *Lancet*, **2**, 477–80

20. Finland, M., Jones, W. F. and Barnes, M. W. (1959). Occurrence of serious bacterial infections since introduction of antibacterial agents. *J. Am. Med. Assoc.*, **170**, 2188–97

21. Smith, I. M. (1980). Common infections in the elderly diabetic. *Geriatrics*, **35(8)**, 55–8

22. Wilson, W. E. C., Kirkpatrick, C. H. and Talmadge, D. W. (1965). Suppression of immunologic responsiveness in uraemia. *Ann. Intern. Med.*, **62**, 1–14

23. Slade, M. S., Simmons, R. L. and Yunis, E. (1975). Immuno-depression after major surgery in normal patients. *Surgery*, **78(3)**, 363–72

24. Likhite, V. V. (1976). Immunologic impairment and susceptibility to infection after splenectomy. *J. Am. Med. Assoc.*, **236**, 1376–7

25. Schrieber, A. D. (1977). Clinical immunology of corticosteroids. In: Schwartz R. S. (ed) *Progress in Immunology*. p. 103. (New York: Grune and Stratton)

26. McGillan, J. and Phair, J. (1979). Polymorphonuclear leucocyte adherence to nylon. Effect of oral corticosteroids. *Infect. Immun.*, **26**, 542–6

27. Burston, G. R. and Moore-Smith, B. (1970). Occult surgical emergencies in the elderly. *Br. J. Clin. Pract.*, **24(6)**, 239–43

28. Cohen, J. (1984). Infection in the compromised host. *Med. Int.* **2(3)**, 123–9

29. Hay, R. J. (1984). Systemic fungal infections and therapy. *Med. Int.*, **2(3)**, 111–17

Index